REIKI HEALING FOR BEGINNERS

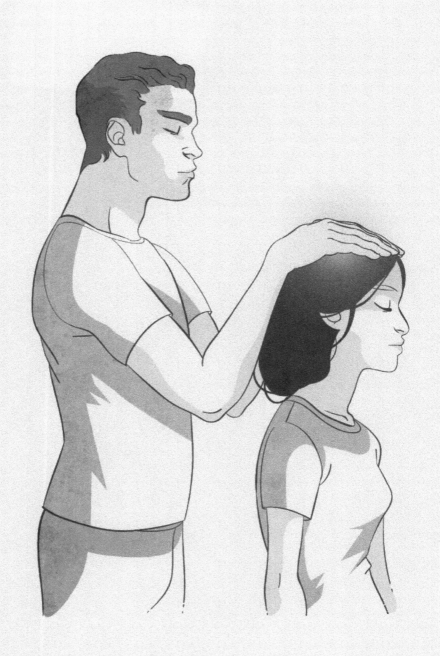

Reiki
Healing

FOR BEGINNERS

The Practical Guide with
Remedies for 100+ Ailments

KAREN FRAZIER

ALTHEA
PRESS

Illustrations © Gloria Pizzilli, 2018

ISBN: Print 978-1-64152-115-4 | eBook 978-1-64152-116-1

For my dad

CONTENTS

INTRODUCTION

Last month, I taught a first-degree Reiki class to a group in Portland, Oregon. Near the end of the class, we engaged in a group practice session, where all of the new Reiki practitioners gathered around one of their classmates and offered hands-on Reiki healing. Each took turns on the Reiki table that day, being the one healed, and I could feel the love and intent flowing between people who had only met that morning at the start of class.

When it was Cassie's turn on the table, something magical happened. As her classmates channeled Reiki energy to her, she began to cry and say, "Thank you, thank you," over and over again. It was a powerful moment of healing none of us will soon forget.

This is why I practice and teach Reiki. By channeling Reiki energy, soul connections are made and lives are powerfully changed.

My first Reiki experience is one I discuss frequently. It was during a difficult period when I lived deeply in the practical world, not really believing there was much more to this universe than what we experience with our five senses. At the time, I had a severe sore throat that had hung on for weeks, impervious to any medical intervention. Finally, in desperation, I went to what I thought was a medical doctor who also offered herbal remedies. It was worth a try, I decided.

What occurred was not what I expected. She was indeed a medical doctor, and she did indeed also offer herbal medicines. But she was a Reiki practitioner, energy healer, and crystal healer as well. Instead of giving me herbs, she laid me on a table, arranged some crystals around me (as I inwardly rolled my eyes), and placed her hands on me in various positions. I was suffused with warmth. And then something gave, and I started to sob uncontrollably.

I continued to cry on and off for three days. But my sore throat went away, and while I get an occasional sore throat from time to time, I've never had one of that intensity or duration again. Likewise, once I'd stopped crying, I felt fantastic. This was the impetus for all that came after it in my life—my exploration of energy healing, crystal energy, Reiki healing, and metaphysics. It was the start of a spiritual journey that has changed my belief system and my life in wondrous ways.

Today, I choose to share what I have discovered on my journey with willing souls who are also seeking something different on their life's path. I offer others tools for empowerment, healing, and self-discovery.

Regardless of where you are on your path, this book is for you. It offers a primer on one of my favorite tools of empowerment, Reiki, a universal healing energy that has the capacity to change lives and, I believe, to change the energy of the planet and the universe in positive ways.

However, before we get to healing the entire universe with Reiki energy, it starts with you. In this book, I give you tools to get started with Reiki, recounting the history of Reiki, sharing with you how to become attuned to and use the energy, and offering you information about how to use Reiki for yourself and others to bring about healing that serves the highest and greatest good. If you're looking for an easy and understandable plan for becoming attuned to and channeling Reiki energy, this is it. We'll explore the common principles and practices of Reiki, and then look at various applications for correcting energetic imbalances that can cause physical, mental, and emotional issues.

I'm honored you are allowing me to share this part of your healing path. Reiki has changed my life, and it can change yours, as well. Namaste (the light in me acknowledges the light in you). I wish you wisdom on your journey.

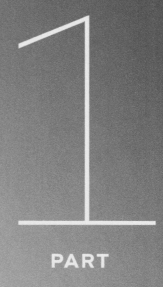

PART

Reiki Basics

1

Introduction to Reiki

Reiki is an ancient healing energy. While it has likely been around since the beginning of time, in the West the story we hear of its origins centers on the legend shared by Madam Hawayo Takata, a Hawaiian Reiki master who brought Reiki from Japan to the Western world. It is Madam Takata who is responsible for the spread of Usui Ryoho Reiki (Usui Reiki) in the West, and Reiki practitioners who have trained here can trace their lineage back to and through her. She taught the history as an oral tradition, so it is sometimes difficult to differentiate between fact and legend. Where possible, I have tried to note which is which.

Origins

All Western Reiki masters are required to teach their first-degree students the history of Reiki, tracing it back through Madam Takata and her master, Dr. Chujiro Hayashi, to his master and teacher, Dr. Mikao Usui. (I'll explain what the degrees mean in chapter 2.) For Western Reiki practitioners, the story begins with Dr. Usui, although sources suggest Reiki was practiced in Japan before Dr. Usui developed his system.

In his book *An Evidence-Based History of Reiki*, William Lee Rand of the International Center for Reiki Training notes that when Dr. Usui's Reiki journey began, there were at least four other types of Reiki being practiced in Japan. So, while the origins of this ancient healing energy practice reach to before our story begins, Western Reiki, also known as Usui Ryoho Reiki, all starts with Mikao Usui and a 21-day meditation on Japan's Mount Kurama.

MIKAO USUI

Mikao Usui (also known as Usui Sensei, "sensei" meaning teacher) was born on August 15, 1865, in Gifu Prefecture (near Nagoya), Japan. Dr. Usui was born into a wealthy Buddhist family, and he traveled extensively for his education, including trips to China and Europe. He studied religion, medicine, divination, and psychology. Throughout his life, Dr. Usui also worked many jobs.

In his personal and spiritual life, Dr. Usui sought answers to some of life's deepest questions. He spent many years in pursuit of a state of consciousness known as An-shin Ritus-mei, which is a deep state of peace and purpose. Pursuing this state, Dr. Usui learned Zen Buddhist practices, including Zazen meditation, at a monastery. Wishing to deepen his practice in order to reach An-shin Ritus-mei, in 1922 Dr. Usui undertook a 21-day meditation and fasting trip to Mount Kurama.

Some Reiki masters suggest that as part of his meditation, Dr. Usui stood under a waterfall on the mountain and allowed it to fall on his head to activate his Crown chakra. According to Madam Takata's oral history, Dr. Usui meditated continuously, and, for each day, he tossed one stone off the mountain. When he no longer had any stones, he knew he had completed his 21 days of meditation.

Legend holds that at midnight on the twenty-first day, Dr. Usui felt light enter his mind through the top of his head, and he lost consciousness. When he awoke several hours later, he was forever changed. He felt vital and alive in a way he hadn't before, despite fasting for 21 days. And he felt his normal consciousness had been replaced with a deep spirituality.

According to legend, Dr. Usui raced down the mountain to share his experience with his Zen master. In his haste, he stubbed his toe on a rock, and when he instinctively grabbed his foot with his hands, it was miraculously healed. When he stopped to eat and rest in a village, the girl who was serving him his meal had a toothache. Dr. Usui placed his hands on her face, and her swelling and pain eased. When he returned to the Zen monastery, Dr. Usui found the abbot in bed with a severe bout of arthritis; Dr. Usui placed his hands on the abbot, who was miraculously healed. These are known in legend as the miracles of Reiki. It is said because of these events, Dr. Usui understood he had received a healing gift, which he called Reiki, the Japanese word for universal life force.

Historical fact picks up where legend ends. While Dr. Usui's experience on Mount Kurama is unsubstantiated information and is therefore considered legend, what is known is that after his experience, Dr. Usui was greatly changed. He moved to Tokyo and began offering Reiki classes and treatments, developing a system for the practices of using Reiki energy. He spent the rest of his life teaching and healing with Reiki. He died on March 9, 1926, in Fukuyama, Japan, but not before meeting and training Dr. Chujiro Hayashi.

CHUJIRO HAYASHI

Chujiro Hayashi was born on September 15, 1880, in Tokyo, Japan. He graduated from the Imperial Japanese Naval Academy with a medical degree in 1902 and became a naval physician. He learned about Reiki from some of his fellow medical professionals who had trained with Dr. Usui. Intrigued, Hayashi began studying Reiki with Dr. Usui in 1925.

Dr. Usui asked Dr. Hayashi to carry on his teachings by establishing a clinic in Tokyo, which he did. It was in Dr. Hayashi's Tokyo clinic that Hawayo Takata started her Reiki training. According to Takata's oral legend, after she returned to Hawaii, Dr. Hayashi visited her in 1937, and she continued her studies. He stayed for several months, teaching Madam Takata. When he returned to Japan in February 1938, however, the Japanese naval authority officials asked Dr. Hayashi to provide information about Hawaii, which he refused to do, and they branded him a spy. To avoid further trouble with his government, Dr. Hayashi died by ritual suicide, seppuku, on May 11, 1940. That Dr. Hayashi performed the ritual of seppuku as an act of honor is an historical fact. The rest is based in legend, and it is unknown if his suicide was for the reason the legend states or for some other reason.

HAWAYO TAKATA

Hawayo Takata was born on the island of Kauai in the territory of Hawaii on December 24, 1900. According to her own account, Takata suffered from abdominal pain, a lung condition, and mental health issues that led to a nervous breakdown. While traveling in Japan for a family matter, Takata was diagnosed with gallstones, asthma, appendicitis, and a tumor, and she was scheduled for surgery. Instead of seeking medical treatment, however, Takata sought Reiki healing from Dr. Hayashi. She was impressed with the results and decided to learn the technique herself.

After spending time in Japan and Hawaii learning Reiki from Dr. Hayashi, Madam Takata developed a system (based on Dr. Usui's and Dr. Hayashi's system) of practicing Reiki, providing healing throughout the United States. In 1970, she also developed a system of teaching new Reiki masters, charging $10,000 for the weekend training because she believed Reiki deserved respect and should never be practiced or taught for free. Madam Takata insisted her students memorize the Reiki system, teaching it as an oral tradition. She cautioned practitioners and masters against providing written materials, such as symbols, hand positions, or even a written history.

In all, Madam Takata trained and attuned 22 Reiki masters. It is her system that is the basis for all Western practices of Usui Reiki, although it has evolved as times have changed. Today, most Reiki masters have done away with the exorbitant fee, and most feel it is appropriate to share Reiki in writing, since both Dr. Usui and Dr. Hayashi provided written materials to their students.

Madam Takata practiced Reiki for more than 40 years. It is because she brought Reiki to the West that this healing practice is known and available outside of Japan.

What Reiki Can Do for You

From Madam Takata's 22 Reiki masters have come thousands of practitioners throughout the Western world practicing Usui Ryoho Reiki. Today, Usui Reiki practitioners trace their Reiki lineage back through their Reiki masters to those who trained and attuned them, going all the way back through Madam Takata and Chujiro Hayashi to Mikao Usui himself. There are hundreds, if not thousands, of Reiki master-teachers across all continents who train and attune new Reiki practitioners, sharing the traditions, history, and practices of this form of energy healing.

HOW REIKI WORKS

No one knows exactly how Reiki works, but many people have experienced its healing power. One possible explanation is the principle of entrainment.

When two oscillating bodies (those that move back and forth or sway) are near each other, they tend to lock into phase (meaning sway at the same frequency) and oscillate in harmony. This occurs due to a law of physics called entrainment, which was initially discovered in the seventeenth century. A Dutch scientist named Christiaan Huygens noticed that when he put two clocks with pendulums close to each other on a wall, they eventually locked into phase, and the pendulums began to swing at the same rate.

Entrainment comes into play in most forms of energy healing, such as crystal and sound healing and hands-on healing like Reiki. When certain energies are in proximity to the human body, the body starts to vibrate in the same frequency as that energy, due to entrainment. People have studied Reiki practitioners during a session and found that their hands emit an energy frequency between 7 Hz and 10 Hz, which is a frequency associated with physical healing.

During a Reiki session, energy flows from the practitioner. Being attuned to Reiki energy by a Reiki master enables Reiki practitioners to align with this energy so it flows freely through their body and into the subject. In this way, the two entrain to bring about healing of the body, mind, and spirit. Therefore, Reiki practitioners aren't actually healers in the traditional sense of the word. A Reiki practitioner is not healing their client. Instead, they are serving as a channel for the healing energy of Reiki. The subject draws the energy the practitioner channels into themselves, and it flows where needed to serve the highest and greatest good.

THE FIVE PRINCIPLES OF REIKI

In his practice, Mikao Usui established the five principles of Reiki that are still used today by Usui Reiki practitioners and masters worldwide. All Reiki practitioners learn the five principles of Reiki in their first-degree lessons. These are the five principles of Reiki:

Just for today, I will not worry.

Just for today, I will not anger.

Just for today, I will do my work honestly.

Just for today, I will be grateful for my many blessings.

Just for today, I will be kind to my neighbor and every living thing.

I recommend meditating on these principles daily. I do so in the morning and the evening, and occasionally even throughout the day when I'm feeling out of balance.

While you may not hit the target of living every single principle every single day, the value is in the awareness and effort to make these principles guiding principles in your life. Continued meditation on these principles can help you move toward integrating them as a regular part of your daily life.

You don't need to memorize the exact wording. In fact, you'll find the same ideas written in many different ways. However, in all cases the meaning is the same:

Try not to worry.

Be slow to anger.

Live with truth and integrity.

Live with gratitude.

Live with kindness and compassion.

If you fall short one day, remember this: Every day, and indeed every moment, is the opportunity to start fresh in bringing these principles into your life. Be as kind to yourself as you would be to others as you integrate these principles into your daily way of living.

HEALING DEFINED

Before discussing the ways in which Reiki energy can benefit you and others, it's important to define healing. Many people misunderstand healing, believing the only way one can heal is to completely rid themselves of symptoms. However, I'm not talking just about removing symptoms when I discuss healing, although symptoms may, indeed, disappear. Instead, by healing I mean the person receiving the energy will move into alignment with that which serves their highest and greatest good.

In some cases, this may mean symptoms or conditions disappear. In other cases, it may have to do with physical, emotional, or spiritual shifts that serve the subject's greatest good to align them with their life's purpose. For example, in my first experience with Reiki, while the disappearance of my sore throat was a benefit of the Reiki treatment, the true healing that occurred was that the energy of my Throat chakra was unblocked and I was able to speak and share my truth about certain circumstances in my life for the first time. That was the true healing that occurred. Reiki continues to serve my highest and greatest good as a teacher, energy healer, writer, and communicator.

HOW REIKI CAN HELP

As you can see, while many people view Reiki as a hands-on energetic modality to bring about physical healing, it serves other important purposes as well.

Reiki can:

- Remove energetic blockages that keep you from moving forward on your life's path
- Help resolve emotional or spiritual issues, such as grief, resentment, or poor self-esteem (among others)

- Balance energy flowing through your energetic systems, which include your chakras, meridians, and aura (discussed in chapter 3)

- Help you find solutions to long-standing issues by offering energetic assistance

- Provide energetic support for physical, spiritual, and emotional issues

- Provide energetic support and healing for animals

- Provide energetic support and healing for the planet or people after natural disasters or traumatic events

- Empower you to live your life in service of your highest and greatest good

How to Use This Book

To channel Reiki energy, you must be attuned to it by a Reiki master-teacher, who can provide teaching and attunements to Usui Reiki in person or at a distance. This book is intended as a supplement to your training with your Reiki master-teacher, who will provide the teachings of and attunements to first, second, and third degree. This book cannot attune you, nor is it meant as a substitute for traditional Reiki training.

What this book provides is easy-to-understand and easy-to-follow information organized in a logical progression that can help you learn how to use Reiki in personal or professional practice. It offers information about the healing and practical applications of Reiki. However, you are still responsible for receiving the appropriate training and attunements and setting up, conducting, and documenting any Reiki business practices according to the laws of where you live and practice.

In part 2, I provide information about the basic hand positions of a hands-on Reiki session for channeling Reiki to others, practicing self-healing, and offering quick sessions when you don't have time for a full hands-on session. After you've learned and practiced the basic hand positions and learned about the Reiki symbols and their use in both hands-on and distance healing, you'll learn about common physical, emotional, mental, and spiritual ailments in part 3. I've chosen the ailments that appear because they are among the most frequent people ask me about as an energy healer and Reiki master-teacher, and I've found energy healing practices have been valuable in helping resolve them or balance the energies involved. For each of these, I'll offer specific information about applying Reiki in person and/or at a distance to help balance the energies that contribute to these ailments.

I am not a medical doctor. The discussion in the chapters that follow is not intended to diagnose any condition or to replace appropriate medical treatment. Likewise, it's essential that you don't diagnose clients yourself, and you always encourage your subjects to seek diagnosis and treatment of all conditions from a qualified medical professional. Your Reiki work with each subject is intended to supplement appropriate diagnosis and care, and this book is offered as a great resource to help you do so. It can help you choose specific Reiki practices, hand positions, and intentions to facilitate healing.

Learning Reiki

I regularly hold classes and offer individual sessions to teach the various degrees of Reiki. My classes and sessions can have anywhere from a single person to 20 people (in one case, a class I taught at a conference with two other Reiki masters had about 50, which is highly unusual). For the most part, I teach my classes in person, although I also do work with students via Skype or video conference. In whatever manner I wind up working with my students, though, the most important thing to me is that I provide them with a solid foundation to understand Reiki, its history and practices, and how to move forward as a confident, compassionate, and powerful Reiki practitioner. When you seek your Reiki teacher, this should be their goal as well.

You and Your Teacher

There are hundreds, if not thousands, of Reiki master-teachers (a designation you'll also see called Shinpiden) you can work with, and all of them go about teaching and attuning their students in slightly different ways. Some only work with their students at a distance, some insist on working with students in person, and some use a combination of both. Some never interact with their students at all, instead offering an online course and then providing a distance attunement. There are even Reiki master-teachers who attune their students while providing no other training or information, assuming their students can rely on books like this one to learn the basics.

In fact, there's not really any "right" way to teach Reiki. While Madam Takata established rigorous requirements for her initiates and how they were to teach and attune others to Usui Ryoho Reiki, as generations of Reiki master-teachers have descended from Madam Takata's original 22, practices in teaching and attuning have changed. The vast majority of Reiki master-teachers share certain elements with students, such as the history, the hand positions, and the techniques, but how teachers go about this varies from person to person. However, just because these are things master-teachers are "supposed" to cover before attuning their students to Reiki doesn't always mean it happens.

WHAT MAKES A SOLID REIKI CURRICULUM?

To be a confident, compassionate, and competent Reiki practitioner, it's important to receive a solid foundation in the history, principles, and practices of Reiki. Therefore, it is essential to work with a master-teacher who is capable of and willing to provide this solid foundation and background. A good Reiki master-teacher will provide you with different things, depending on the degree of Reiki you are learning, but should always include:

- A written manual outlining the history of Reiki, the appropriate principles for the degree of Reiki you are learning, and the essential tools and knowledge for practicing in that degree (although some Reiki master-teachers don't provide these written materials because they firmly believe, as Madam Takata did, that Reiki should be shared only as an oral tradition)

- A class or one-on-one session where you learn the principles through oral or written communication (in person or at a distance), have the opportunity to practice the associated skills, and have the opportunity to have any and all questions asked and answered

- Clear instructions about how to perform any required elements of your degree of Reiki

- A Reiki attunement that is appropriate for the degree of Reiki you are learning

- Supplemental materials to reinforce key concepts, as needed

- The potential for ongoing mentorship, as needed

If a master-teacher can provide even more background information to help you be a stronger, more knowledgeable, and more confident energy healer, even better. For example, in my Reiki classes, along with the basics, I also provide information about energy healing in general, the human energy anatomy, general principles of energy healing, and supplemental energy healing practices (such as sound healing, crystals, and aromatherapy). While these things aren't required, they do enhance your knowledge and credibility as a Reiki practitioner and enable you to provide your clients with a powerful healing experience.

FINDING THE RIGHT MASTER-TEACHER

In general, the quality of the master-teacher you select influences the type of Reiki practitioner you become. As with any other institution, you'll find Reiki master-teachers with varying degrees of competence, experience, standards, values and ethics, and accountability. Therefore, it's in your best interests (and in the best interests of the institution of Reiki as a whole) to find a master-teacher and mentor who maintains the highest possible standards and levels of accountability and ethics.

With so many options for learning and being attuned to Reiki, from static online classes that are a series of articles followed by a distance attunement, to one-on-one hands-on mentoring and coaching, it isn't necessarily *how* you learn Reiki that matters as long as you find a master-teacher who will provide a solid foundation that best suits your schedule, budget, and mentorship needs. It's also helpful to find a master-teacher whose teaching techniques suit your learning style and one with whom you "vibe" and feel comfortable.

For my Reiki students, my intent is to provide ongoing mentorship from the moment they set foot in my first-degree Reiki class throughout the rest of their time working with Reiki, even up to and through the master-teacher degree. I keep lines of communication open with my students throughout their lifetime (or mine), working with them in person, online, on the phone, and in social-networking groups, such as through Facebook. I encourage (but don't require) my students to stay in contact with me and with the network of other Reiki practitioners with whom I have worked. I feel this is the gold standard of mentorship, and it is one I am delighted to offer because I believe spreading Reiki and energy healing is such a deeply humbling honor and responsibility. If you can find a master-teacher who feels a similar level of responsibility toward their students, grab hold with both hands, because that relationship will serve you well as you practice all degrees of Reiki.

Distance or in Person?

You'll find some Reiki master-teachers and practitioners believe you should never work with a student at a distance, insisting on only in-person interaction. And while I definitely prefer to work with my students in person and recognize the benefits of doing so, I also realize it is possible to provide excellent training and mentorship at a distance. Therefore, what you choose is totally up to you.

Qualifications

The qualifications your Reiki master-teacher needs are:

- Being trained in and attuned to first-, second-, and third- (master-teacher) degree Reiki
- Being able to show you certificates documenting their qualifications
- Being able to offer you documentation of their Reiki lineage, starting with themselves and extending backward through all teachers to Mikao Usui

Questions to Ask

When vetting potential master-teachers, ask the following questions and consider how their answers suit your needs.

1. How long have you practiced Reiki? What are your approximate dates of training and attunement to each degree of Reiki? When did you become a master-teacher?

2. What can I expect if I pursue Reiki training and attunement with you?

3. How many students have you trained and attuned?

4. What information do you provide before each degree of attunement?

5. Do you prefer to teach in person or at a distance? What are the benefits of your way of teaching?

6. What ongoing education or support do you offer your students after each degree of training?

7. Do you belong to any organizations or trade groups as a Reiki master-teacher? Which ones?

8. What written materials and documentation will you provide me?

9. What is your personal philosophy of Reiki and energy healing?

10. Do you have a background in other forms of energy healing? Which ones?

11. Do you pursue any other religious or theological viewpoint in conjunction with your Reiki, and if so, is it part of your personal training and philosophy? How does it change or affect how you teach and practice Reiki?

12. Do you actively practice Reiki on clients, or do you strictly teach and provide attunements?

13. What is the maximum number of people you allow in each Reiki class?

14. Are you willing to supply references?

A Typical Reiki Class and Attunement

While it varies from master to master, there are some general things you may expect as you embark on your Reiki journey with a class and an attunement. An attunement is the process in which your Reiki master-teacher will align you with whatever degree of Reiki you are working with so you can channel it.

THE CLASS

Most instructors offer anywhere from one to eight (or more) hours of classroom instruction, in person or online, for each degree of Reiki. In the class, you may be the only participant, or there may be many other students. Your master-teacher will likely provide you with a manual outlining all of the material they are teaching for that degree (I provide mine as an electronic file my students can download) and handouts for supplementary material, if needed. They will also provide instruction for the degree of Reiki you are learning, either as a lecture or as online written content. In person, they will provide you with the opportunity for hands-on practice and answer any questions you may have.

Most master-teachers charge a fee, although some may not. Fees vary depending on the type and length of class, the number of students, and other factors. Group lessons will cost less than private sessions, and remote lessons may be less than in-person sessions.

YOUR ATTUNEMENT

Your Reiki attunement aligns you to the energy in the degree of Reiki you are learning. Each succeeding degree of Reiki attunes you to a higher level of the energy and to the energy of the symbols (if any) used in that degree. (To learn about the symbols, see page 37.) Only a Reiki master-teacher (Shinpiden) who has been attuned to third-degree Reiki can attune people to all degrees of Reiki energy.

Toward the end of the session, your instructor will perform your attunement to the Reiki energy. In large on-site classes, you will sit in a circle in Gassho (a meditative Reiki posture; you place your hands together in prayer position in front of you with your middle fingers gently touching) with your eyes closed while your instructor attunes the students one at a time. In such sessions, attunement for each student takes about five minutes.

In an individual in-person class, your instructor will have you sit with your eyes closed in Gassho as they attune you. If your attunement is at a distance, you will contact your Reiki master-teacher at a preset time. They will instruct you to sit comfortably at the designated time in a quiet area, away from disturbances. Plan for about 15 minutes for a distance attunement.

You must be attuned to a degree of Reiki (first, second, or third) to be able to channel the Reiki energy at that level. You must be attuned in order, as well. That is, you can't be attuned to second-degree Reiki until you have been attuned to first-degree Reiki, and you can't be attuned to master-teacher degree (third) until you have been attuned to first- and second-degree Reiki.

Some master-teachers attune to a single degree of Reiki at a time, with a period between attunements to allow the practitioner to get used to working with that degree of the Reiki energy and have the opportunity to do so. Other master-teachers may attune their students to more than one of the degrees at the same time, or even to all three degrees at once, depending on the circumstances, the needs of the student, and the curriculum. For example, in some cases, when a student has a strong need to perform distance Reiki such as for an ill relative who lives across the country, I may teach and attune both first- and second-degree Reiki at the same time.

There is no right or wrong way to do this. What's important is that the timing of the attunements serves the highest and greatest good of you and those you are working with.

With that being said, there is a timeline I generally follow. I like to allow space between attunements so my student can adapt to the new Reiki energy and become a competent and confident practitioner before moving on to the next degree. When I don't follow this timeline, it is usually because my student has specific needs, or I intuitively feel I need to follow a different schedule. In general, this is the timeline I follow:

- Start with a first-degree Reiki attunement. I allow the practitioner to work with the energy for three to six months (or longer). At minimum, I try to keep 21 days between a first- and second-degree attunement to allow for the 21-day detoxification process (see page 24). This detox will occur after each degree of attunement.

- After three to six months, I provide second-degree Reiki training and attunement. I allow the practitioner to work with this energy for about six months to a year so the student truly understands the Reiki energy before teaching it to others. At a minimum, I try to allow 21 days between this and the next degree.

- About a year (or longer) from first-degree Reiki, I provide third-degree (master-teacher) Reiki energy to students who wish to pursue it at this level.

While these are general guidelines, sometimes this timeline is compressed, and other times it is lengthened based on the needs of my students. You'll find other teachers who do this differently.

Before Your Attunement
In the 24 hours before your attunement, it is helpful (but not necessary) to take the following steps to help you prepare:

- Get plenty of sleep the night before.
- Refrain from using intoxicants for at least 24 hours before your attunement.
- Drink plenty of water and eat light, nutritious foods.
- Meditate in the morning before your attunement.

THE THREE PILLARS OF REIKI

In second-degree Reiki, as practitioners deepen their practice, they learn the three pillars of Reiki. These are the three practices that serve as the basis for a Reiki session.

The First Pillar: Gassho

Pronounced *gash-SHOW*, Gassho is a meditative Reiki practice that means "two hands coming together." In Gassho, you place your hands together in prayer position in front of you, with your middle fingers gently touching. Dr. Usui taught his students to use Gassho as a daily meditative practice, advising them to focus on where the middle fingertips touch, gently bringing focus back to this point if the mind wanders. This is an excellent way to begin every Reiki session.

The Second Pillar: Reiji Ho

Pronounced *ray-GEE-hoe*, Reiji Ho means "methods of indication of Reiki power." It involves a series of rituals to strengthen your practice. The methods use the Reiki symbols, which practitioners learn in second-degree Reiki. Many practitioners use Reiji Ho as part of their healing sessions, in place of or as a supplement to the hand positions. To perform Reiji Ho:

1. Stand at the client's feet with hands in Gassho and eyes closed.

2. Mentally draw the symbol Hon Sha Ze Sho Nen (HSZN), mentally intone its name, and ask for Reiki energy to flow.

3. Do this three times.

4. Visualize the symbol Sei He Ki (SHK), saying its name mentally three times.

5. Visualize the symbol Cho Ku Rei (CKR), saying its name mentally three times.

6. Ask Reiki energy to balance your subject.

7. Keeping your hands in Gassho, move them up to and in front of your third eye (forehead) and ask them to guide your hands to where the Reiki energy is most needed. Follow this guidance without agenda or personal desires.

The Third Pillar: Chiryo

Pronounced *chi-RYE-oh*, this pillar means "treatment." Chiryo serves as an alternative to the traditional Reiki hand positions. In Reiki practice, the treatment involves holding your hands over the Crown chakra until you are guided to move. Once you receive such guidance, you may move your hands to the desired position for three to five minutes, or until you receive guidance to move again.

In between hand positions, return to the client's Crown chakra and wait again for guidance, moving when intuition suggests you do. Do this until the session feels complete.

During Your Attunement

My students report various experiences during their attunement (both in person and at a distance). You may experience some, all, or none of the following:

- Seeing swirling lights
- Feeling a deep sense of peace and joy
- Noticing an emotional release
- Feeling your hands "turn on"—that is, you suddenly notice heat or tingling in your hands
- Feeling flushes of warmth throughout your body
- Feeling intense emotion of any type

Any and all of these reactions are normal, as is not experiencing anything. The trick is to allow the experience and accept it for what it is.

During an in-person attunement, you will feel your Reiki master-teacher moving around you. They may touch you, draw symbols on you using a fingertip or in the air near you, and may physically reposition your hands. Some Reiki master-teachers also use a process called the violet breath, which involves blowing a breath into your hands. I don't use this in my attunements, but I know many master-teachers who do. My master-teacher used it, and because I wasn't aware it was coming, I was slightly startled. So just be aware that for some Reiki master-teachers, this is an important part of the attunement ceremony.

After the ceremony, drink a glass of cold water to help ground you. Discuss any unusual experiences, observations, or questions with your master-teacher.

After Your Attunement

After you are attuned, you will experience a 21-day detoxification process. During this time, you may notice changes in your physical, emotional, mental, or spiritual states. You may notice some mild physical symptoms, such as a runny nose or congestion, and you may also find you are more or less emotional than usual. You may also have disturbed or deeper sleep, vivid dreams, or notice your hands will suddenly "turn on" (tingle or feel warm) for no apparent reason. All of these reactions are normal.

During this time, give yourself daily self-Reiki treatments (see chapter 4), drink plenty of water, try to get lots of sleep, and meditate daily. This will help you as you move through the 21-day cleansing process.

Degrees of Reiki

Throughout this book, I've referred to the three degrees of Usui Ryoho Reiki: first, second, and third (master-teacher). The following is a brief outline of what each degree represents.

FIRST-DEGREE REIKI

The following elements comprise first-degree Reiki training and attunement:

- History of Reiki (based on legend and fact)
- Five principles of Reiki
- Reiki hand positions for healing self and others
- Hands-on Reiki practice
- Instruction in how to provide hands-on healing sessions to friends, family, and self
- Attunement to the first-degree Reiki energy

After completing first-degree Reiki training and attunement, practitioners are able to channel Reiki energy in person to others via hands-on treatment.

IF YOU WANT TO SET UP REIKI AS A BUSINESS, KEEP THESE THINGS IN MIND

In the United States, the Health Insurance Portability and Accountability Act of 1996 (HIPAA) applies to any type of health-care provider, including energy healers. It mandates certain data privacy and security provisions to safeguard medical information. You will need to ensure you are compliant with all HIPAA requirements.

- Client confidentiality is essential and expected. Do not disclose any client information, no matter how minor, without written permission.

- You will likely need liability insurance to protect yourself. There are a number of organizations that offer liability insurance for Reiki practitioners at reasonable rates.

- Familiarize yourself with local, regional, and national laws governing energy healing practitioners in your area, as well as with laws governing the establishment of businesses. For example, laws in the United States and Great Britain are vastly different regarding who can practice Reiki as a business, and business laws may vary from town to town. Make sure you also have the proper insurance and licenses.

- You will need to document everything. Keep files on all of your clients, use the appropriate intake paperwork, and document your sessions.

- Have all clients sign an informed consent waiver before any treatment begins.

- Reiki training does not make you a medical practitioner. Therefore, by law you cannot diagnose. Never diagnose any of your clients with anything, ever, and never contradict a diagnosis from a medical professional or tell a client to stop an existing medical treatment.

- If you are working as adjunct therapy for a medical condition with a licensed medical professional, it is in your client's and your best interests to have a signed note of approval, or at least acknowledgment of treatment from that professional—or, if possible, a referral.

SECOND-DEGREE REIKI

Second-degree Reiki training and attunement consists of the following:

- Training in the three pillars of Reiki
- Instruction on how to perform intuitive Reiki using the three pillars (as opposed to using only the hand positions)
- Instruction in and attunement to the three second-degree Reiki symbols required to channel second-degree Reiki and offer distance Reiki sessions
- Instruction about distance healing techniques that enable you to send Reiki healing across space and time
- Other advanced Reiki techniques, at the discretion of the master-teacher
- Information about sending Reiki to situations and to the planet
- Ethics of distance healing
- In some cases, information about setting up a Reiki practice, necessary paperwork, etc.
- Attunement to second-degree Reiki energy

THIRD-DEGREE REIKI (MASTER-TEACHER/SHINPIDEN)

This is the essential training that allows you to teach and attune others to all three degrees of Reiki. Third-degree Reiki instruction includes the following:

- Instruction in and attunement to the Reiki master symbol
- Instruction in and attunement to other symbols, at the master-teacher's discretion
- Instruction in teaching and attuning others to all three degrees of Reiki

- Instruction in standards, practices, and ethics for Reiki master-teachers
- Attunement to third-degree (master-teacher/Shinpiden) Reiki energy
- Other instruction, at the master-teacher's discretion

After attunement to master-teacher degree Reiki, you will be able to teach others and attune them to all three degrees of Reiki.

10 Tips for Starting Your Reiki Journey

If you'd like to get started on the empowering journey of becoming an attuned Reiki practitioner of any degree, consider the following tips:

1. If you've never experienced a hands-on Reiki session before, it's good to have one before you learn Reiki yourself. This will help you understand what others will experience when you provide Reiki.

2. Think about your time, needs, and budget. Then you can contact a Reiki organization, like the International Association of Reiki Professionals, to find a Reiki master-teacher near you.

3. Ask others for recommendations about Reiki master-teachers who share your values and meet your mentorship and learning needs.

4. Be sure you chat with your Reiki master-teacher ahead of time to ensure it's a good match. Learning and attunement to Reiki is a deeply personal journey, and you'll want to find an instructor you "vibe" with.

5. You don't need to have the same Reiki master-teacher for every degree. In fact, I have two separate master-teachers; one met one set of needs for me, and the other met another.

6. Don't rush it. Allow yourself the time to learn and get used to the Reiki energy, and practice working with it before moving up degrees.

7. If you plan to channel Reiki to others, you'll want a good Reiki treatment table for freedom of movement and ease in achieving the correct hand positions. You can find affordable, high-quality massage tables online for under $100. I have a lovely portable table I keep in my office that I can take with me when I teach classes elsewhere.

8. Consider joining a formal organization or an informal group for support, advice, fellowship, and ongoing information about Reiki. (Even if I didn't teach and attune you to Reiki, you are welcome to join my Facebook group, the SHARe Reiki Community; see the Resources section at the end of this book.)

9. Become a Reiki sponge. Give yourself Reiki as often as possible, seek Reiki from others as often as possible, and make use of as many resources as possible to continue to learn and grow as a Reiki practitioner and healer.

10. Utilize the resources found at the end of this book, which provide additional information about setting up a Reiki practice and offer you great books and online sources for learning more.

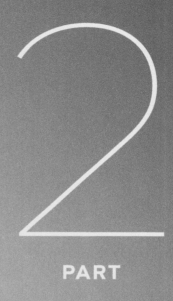

PART

Reiki Healing Techniques

Common Reiki Tools

Reiki is one of many forms of energy healing that work with the human energy anatomy, which is also sometimes called the subtle anatomy. A basic understanding of the subtle anatomy is helpful, because it gives you a better understanding of the work you are doing.

Energy Anatomy

You aren't just a body. You're also mind, emotions, and spirit, and all of these combined make up the whole of you. You can't have one without the others, and it's important for your health and well-being that you seek to balance all four.

Traditional medicine studies the body and, to some extent, the mind and emotions. Each of these elements of you has physical aspects. For example, some of your thoughts and emotions are controlled by chemicals in your body, such as hormones and neurotransmitters.

Energy healing focuses on all four, giving equal importance to the aspects of mind, emotions, and spirit that are not physical, such as your consciousness, intuition, and higher self. Your energy anatomy reflects not only your physical self, but also your spiritual self. It is the intersection between the physical you and the etheric you—the part of you that consists of a web of energy.

Energy healers identify three main aspects of the energy anatomy as follows:

• Your **aura** is the energy field that surrounds your physical body.

• Your **meridians** are energy pathways that run throughout your body—sort of the energetic equivalent of your blood vessels.

• Your **chakras** are swirling wheels of energy that run along your central core and connect your physical self to your higher self. We will focus on the chakras as the main component of energy anatomy when working with Reiki.

Chakras

You have seven main chakras running through your core. Visualize them as colorful swirling wheels or balls of light that run up your spine all the way to the top of your head and carry energy from your etheric self to your physical self.

When your chakras are energetically balanced and operating at optimum efficiency, your life is in balance and so is your spiritual, mental, emotional, and physical health. However, when energy is not balanced in one or more chakras, problems may arise. Imbalances may be caused by excessive energy in a chakra, not enough energy in a chakra, or even a complete blockage of energy in that chakra. In her book *Anatomy of the Spirit,* author Caroline Myss identifies specific physical, mental, emotional, and spiritual issues associated with energetic imbalances in each chakra.

When you channel Reiki energy, you can help rebalance this chakra energy to bring your subjects back to a greater state of physical, spiritual, emotional, and mental balance. Sometimes directing Reiki energy to a specific chakra can quickly help rebalance energies and resolve conditions related to that chakra.

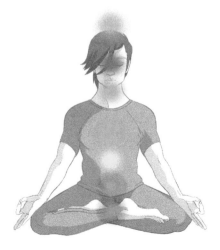

ROOT CHAKRA (FIRST CHAKRA)

The Root chakra, also called Muladhara, is at the base of the spine. Its color is red, and physical issues associated with imbalanced energy here tend to be in the hips, legs, and rectum. Mentally, the Root chakra is the source of emotional well-being, and it is also related to safety, security, loyalty, trust, and connection to the physical world (grounding).

SACRAL CHAKRA (SECOND CHAKRA)

Also known as Svadhisthana, the Sacral chakra is orange. It is located slightly below the navel region. Physically, problems of the intestines and lower back may be related to imbalances here. It is also the seat of personal power and the birthplace of creativity. People with imbalances in this region may also experience issues related to sexuality, prosperity, control, and addiction.

SOLAR PLEXUS CHAKRA (THIRD CHAKRA)

The Solar Plexus chakra, also known as Manipura, is located at the base of the sternum. It is gold or yellow, and the energy here is where you form your personality and develop a sense of self as separate from others (particularly your family or tribe). Imbalances are associated with poor self-esteem and self-worth, feeling like an outsider, lack of willingness to work within social rules, or a lack of personal honor and integrity. Physically, the Solar Plexus chakra is associated with the abdominal organs, the diaphragm, and the middle back.

HEART CHAKRA (FOURTH CHAKRA)

Also called Anahata, the Heart chakra is green and is located in the center of the chest. The Heart chakra serves as the energetic bridge between body and spirit, and it is the seat of love, kindness, and compassion. Issues associated with Heart chakra imbalances include the inability or need to forgive, anger, grief, bitterness, and self-centeredness. Physically, the Heart chakra is associated with the heart, lungs, circulatory system, respiratory system, shoulders, arms, hands, and upper-middle back.

THROAT CHAKRA (FIFTH CHAKRA)

The Throat chakra is blue and located just above the Adam's apple. It's also called Vishuddha. Physically, the Throat chakra is associated with the throat, thyroid, parathyroid, teeth, jaw, and gums, as well as the neck and the lower portion of the face. Problems associated with a Throat chakra imbalance include lack of integrity or truthfulness, the inability to speak out, and issues with creative expression and self-expression.

THIRD EYE CHAKRA (SIXTH CHAKRA)

Also known as Ajna, the Third Eye chakra is indigo or violet. It is in the center of the forehead and is associated with intuition, intellect, spirituality, open-mindedness, and reasoning. Physical issues associated with imbalances here may be in the eyes, ears, head, or brain, and may include mental health problems.

CROWN CHAKRA (SEVENTH CHAKRA)

The Crown chakra, which is just above the crown of the skull, is white or clear, and is also known as Sahasrara. Systemic physical issues and mental illnesses are associated with the Crown chakra. This chakra is also associated with a connection to the divine, ethics and values, and understanding of the greater self as one with the universe.

Reiki Symbols

The traditional Reiki tools are hand positions and symbols. Hand positions are traditional hand placements as taught by Madam Takata that enable you to channel Reiki evenly throughout the body. Symbols are drawn or traced and used to help direct Reiki energy in certain ways. You may also work with other energy healing tools, so understanding them all will help you be a more effective Reiki practitioner.

Beyond first-degree Reiki, you will learn four main Reiki symbols (three in second degree and one in master-teacher degree) that enable you to strengthen and direct your Reiki energy, attune others to Reiki energy, and send Reiki across time and distance so you don't need to conduct hands-on sessions. A Reiki master must attune you to these symbols so you can use them in your Reiki healing sessions. If you have not been attuned to the energy of the symbols, using them will not have the desired effect. To use the symbols, you can activate them in various ways, typically by tracing them on your hands or visualizing them in your mind as you work. Some Reiki masters may also teach and attune you to additional symbols, but they aren't part of the standard practice of Reiki.

SECOND-DEGREE SYMBOLS

In second-degree Reiki, your master-teacher will teach you and attune you to the following three symbols. These symbols unlock the power of second-degree Reiki, helping you focus and strengthen your energy. Once you are attuned to these symbols, you are attuned for life.

Cho Ku Rei (CKR)

Pronounced *CHO-koo-ray*, CKR is the Reiki power symbol. It means "placing the power of the universe here."

- Cho = to remove illusion in order to see truth
- Ku = to penetrate
- Rei = present everywhere, universal

CKR amplifies Reiki energy and activates all other Reiki symbols. When you use the CKR symbol, it can do any of the following:

- Change Reiki energy to second-degree Reiki energy (without it, you are only providing first-degree energy)
- Cut through resistance and release energetic blockages
- Activate other symbols
- Help with the act of dis-creation; that is, it allows you to undo situations you have created energetically
- Help dis-create disease
- Purify energy in a room or space
- Provide protective energy
- Cleanse objects
- Help balance energies
- Strengthen affirmations and visualizations.

These are some of the ways I personally use CKR:

- I trace it on the steering wheel of my car before every trip to balance my car's energy and optimize its performance.
- I trace CKR in the corners of spaces I am visiting, such as hotel rooms or classrooms where I teach, to draw beneficial Reiki energy and provide protection.

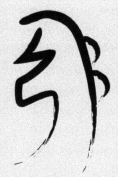

Cho Ku Rei (CKR)

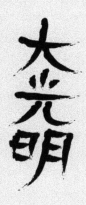

Sei He Ki (SHK)

Hon Sha Ze Sho Nen (HSZN)

Dai Ko Myo (DKM)

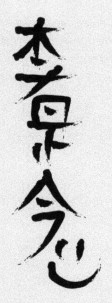

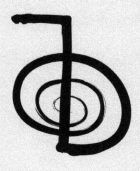

- I use CKR to cleanse my home, tracing it in every corner of every room and over doorways and windows (all entry points to the home) to ensure the energy that enters my home is beneficial and positive.
- I trace the symbol over my food and drink before I consume it.
- I trace it over water and food I feed my plants and my animals to balance their energies as well.
- I use it in conjunction with my personal visualization and affirmations, drawing it before and after each session.

To activate CKR, you must say the name of the symbol (aloud or in your head) three times anytime you draw it.

Sei He Ki (SHK)

Pronounced *say-HAY-kee*, SHK is the Reiki symbol of emotional healing. It means "man and God become one."

- Sei = birth or coming into being
- He Ki = equilibrium or balance

If you're working with a deeply emotional situation, using this symbol can help. It can also help clear emotional and energetic blockages. It's excellent to use in situations where emotions are imbalanced, such as someone grieving deeply. Other uses for this symbol include:

- Clearing energy that is blocked or where there is deep emotional resistance, such as in deeply ingrained habits or long-term problems, including addiction
- Removing obstacles
- Helping unstick relationships where people are deeply entrenched in their own point of view
- Helping process negative emotions
- Bringing calm to volatile situations
- Sparking intuition

- Sparking creativity

- Improving communication

To activate SHK, you must use CKR. To do this, you can create what is commonly known as a Reiki sandwich, where you draw the symbol CKR around SHK on either end: CKR + SHK + CKR. As you draw each symbol mentally or physically, be sure you say the name of each (either aloud or in your head) three times each time you draw it.

Hon Sha Ze Sho Nen (HSZN)

Pronounced *Hon-SHAW-ze-SHOW-nen*, HSZN is the Reiki distance healing symbol. This is the symbol you use to send Reiki to someone at a distance across either space or time. To use HSZN, you must activate it with CKR by bracketing it with the CKR symbol: CKR + HSZN + CKR. While this is sufficient for sending Reiki at a distance, most practitioners use a full Reiki sandwich that incorporates all second-degree symbols, like this:

CKR + SHK + CKR + HSZN + CKR

As you draw each symbol, make sure you say its name mentally or aloud three times.

You can send Reiki across time and distance to yourself or others once you are attuned to second-degree Reiki and these symbols. For example, you can:

- Send healing to someone who needs it

- Send healing to natural disasters or tragic events

- Send healing to the planet

- Send healing to animals that it's best not to touch, such as wild animals

- Send healing to yourself or others in the future for important events, such as a job interview or a major health appointment

- Send Reiki to your pets when you are away so they feel comforted by your presence

When you use the second-degree Reiki symbols to send Reiki energy at a distance, it is important to have permission from your subject, just as you would if you were channeling Reiki in person. If you have been unable to get permission (or if you are sending it to a group or situation), then as you channel the Reiki, intend for it to go to that person or event, and if they don't wish to receive it, intend for the Reiki to go wherever it is most needed to serve the highest and greatest good.

Dai Ko Myo (DKM)

In the master-teacher degree, you will learn and be attuned to the Reiki master symbol, Dai Ko Myo. Pronounced *dye-ko-MEE-oh*, DKM means "bright shining light." Only Reiki masters who have been attuned to the symbol and master-teacher degree Reiki will be able to use this symbol.

DKM represents love, light, and harmony, and is symbolic of the source energy of which we are all made and to which we all return. Using the symbol enables you to channel third-degree Reiki energy and balances all energies: body, mind, emotions, and spirit. It helps integrate the physical with the etheric. You can also use it by itself to replace all of the second-degree symbols. As with other symbols, when you use it, to activate it you must say its name silently or aloud three times as you draw it.

USING THE SYMBOLS

There are many ways you can introduce the symbols to Reiki sessions, such as:

- Drawing them on your hands before channeling Reiki energy
- Drawing them on the body of your subject as you channel Reiki energy
- Visualizing drawing them above the body of your subject and seeing your subject drawing them in as you channel Reiki energy

ACUPUNCTURE AND REIKI

Acupuncture is a form of energy healing that can complement Reiki. In acupuncture, a licensed practitioner places thin needles in meridian points where energy flow may be blocked or overactive to help rebalance energy flow throughout the meridians.

While Reiki flows where it is needed, acupuncture helps release specific points to allow the energy to flow freely. The two therapies work synergistically and can help your clients heal more quickly than using either modality alone.

While it isn't necessary to combine the two, in many cases it benefits your client to take this twofold path. If you plan to practice Reiki, I recommend finding a reputable acupuncturist in your area to whom you can refer clients, if needed. Likewise, your work as a Reiki practitioner may be helpful to some of the acupuncturist's clients, so setting up a mutual referral agreement can benefit everyone involved, especially the clients.

If you do establish a referral relationship, make sure it's with someone you've spent some time with who shares your values and ethics as a healer. It's important that the person to whom you refer your clients shares your same intense focus on kindness, compassion, and providing energy healing that serves the highest and greatest good of your clients.

- Drawing them on a photograph of a Reiki subject at a distance
- Drawing them on written affirmations

When working with the symbols, use your intuition. Ask which symbol will work the best for any given situation and follow what you are intuitively guided to do. Your Reiki master-teacher will also provide specific instruction in using the symbols as you move into the appropriate degree of Reiki.

Meditation

Meditation can help clear your mind, provide balance, and put you in the space for channeling Reiki energy. Dr. Usui recommended meditating in Gassho every day, as well as meditating for a few moments before a session when you channel Reiki. Meditation allows you to tune in to the Reiki energy and clear your mind of any expected outcome. It can also help bring you to a positive, peaceful, and relaxed state of mind in which you are better able to listen to and act on your intuition throughout a Reiki session. I recommend meditating in some way daily to help you stay positive and focused in your work as a Reiki practitioner.

Here's an admission: I used to be terrified of meditation. Back in the day, when I attempted to meditate I always felt it went terribly. I'd try to sit somewhere quietly in the lotus position and clear my mind, but I would quickly become aware my mind wasn't cleared at all. Therefore, I decided, I was a failure at meditation.

Many of my students express similar concerns and difficulties with meditation to me, and I get it. I spent most of my twenties and thirties and part of my forties believing I couldn't meditate. Then I realized that wasn't true; I just hadn't found *my* way to meditate.

While traditional meditation does, indeed, involve sitting and trying to clear your mind (or, in the case of Reiki, sitting in Gassho and focusing on where your middle fingers touch), that's not the only way to meditate. In fact, meditating can be anything that allows you to clear your mind, focus, and move into a more positive space. For me, that's often either movement meditation (I do a form of dance called Nia that is a very meditative experience for me) or listening to music and allowing myself to get carried away in it. For other people, meditation may happen while walking, focusing on breathing, working on a meditative activity such as a craft, or engaging in focused mental activity such as affirmation, visualization, or prayer. It doesn't have to involve sitting in the lotus position and chanting "om" for 20 minutes—although if that works for you, go for it.

I recommend meditating for 20 minutes each day, or as often as you can. I've made it a daily practice, and how I meditate varies depending on what my needs are for that day. Here are some things to try:

• Go for a walk and clear your mind. Breathe deeply and focus on your five senses instead of your thoughts.

• Take a yoga class and focus on your movement and breathing.

• Gaze at a candle or crystal. When your attention wanders, gently bring it back to the focus point.

• Find a guided meditation that speaks to you and listen to that.

• Put on headphones, seek a quiet spot, and listen to music that stirs you. Allow yourself to get lost in the music.

• Speak affirmations, meditate on the five principles of Reiki, or visualize things you'd like to experience or achieve.

• Put on music and dance, allowing yourself to get lost in music and movement.

• Journal.

• Lie quietly and focus on your breathing.

• Chant a mantra that has meaning for you.

If some days it isn't working for you, give yourself a break and return to your meditation practice when you are better able to do so. If 20 minutes seems too long, start with 10 minutes and work your way up. The goal is to take time to focus and disconnect from all of your thoughts, and there's really no wrong way to do it if what you're doing works for you.

Crystals

I could write a whole book about crystals; in fact, I have written a few. I use crystals as part of my everyday practice and also incorporate them into my Reiki classes and channeling sessions.

Crystals are gifts from the Earth that vibrate with a gentle healing energy. I explained earlier how Reiki works by using the principle of entrainment, and crystals work the same way. Each crystal has a vibration that lends itself to various healing energies. I use crystals to unstick static energy, increase vibration, balance chakras, create better energy in spaces, and for dozens of other reasons.

When working with crystals, there are many, many books and websites that can teach you which crystals can help in which situations. I recommend choosing crystals using these sources, as well as by listening intuitively to what crystals you feel lead you to them.

In Reiki sessions, you can use crystals in the following ways:

- Place appropriate crystals around or under your treatment table to help balance energies.
- Place crystals around your healing room to promote positive energy.

- Place crystals on your subject as you channel Reiki. For example, you may wish to place crystals that match the color of each of the chakras over your subject's chakras to help balance them as you channel Reiki energy.

- Use clear quartz to help amplify Reiki energy.

- Use black tourmaline to block negative energy during a Reiki session.

- Use smoky quartz to transmute negative energy into positive energy during a Reiki session.

- Use Apache tears in a Reiki session to help release powerful emotions, such as grief.

- Use rose quartz to facilitate compassion and unconditional love during a session.

- Use a black or red stone to ground yourself after a Reiki session and to ground your subject when they are done with the session.

- Hold clear quartz in your hand and channel Reiki to it, adding a stated intention (such as, "I intend this clear quartz crystal to help balance [subject's name]'s energies for their highest and greatest good"). Then place the quartz on the table.

- Channel Reiki energy to a piece of clear quartz with the intention that it amplify and continue to supply Reiki energy, and then give it to your subject to take with them.

- Meditate with crystals before you channel Reiki.

- Use a crystal of your choice as a surrogate to hold in your hands as you channel distance Reiki.

After using a crystal in a Reiki session, be sure you cleanse it before using it in your next session. To do this, hold the crystal in your hands and channel Reiki to it for two or three minutes.

Essential Oils

Creating a relaxing and pleasant ambience is beneficial to both you and your subject when you channel Reiki. I love to diffuse essential oils in my healing space, both for their pleasant aromas and for their healing properties.

I recommend a simple diffuser in your healing space. Try to find aromas that are pleasant and relaxing, and avoid anything too stimulating (such as cinnamon or peppermint). The goal is to contribute to the relaxing, healing atmosphere. Choose organic essential oils or blends (one of my favorite brands is Edens Garden), and make sure you're using essential oils and not perfume oils.

I also put a few drops each of lavender, tea tree, and orange essential oils in water in a spray bottle and use it to clean my table between clients without harsh chemicals.

Here are a few essential oils to consider:

- Lavender is a relaxing scent that can help balance Third Eye and Heart chakra energies. It has a pleasant, floral aroma, and it's quite affordable.

- Myrrh oil can aid in grounding and balancing the Root chakra.

- Sandalwood has a pleasant, woodsy aroma that can help balance body, mind, and spirit, and also balances the Sacral, Third Eye, and Crown chakras.

- Lemon has an uplifting, cheerful scent that also balances the Solar Plexus chakra.

- Eucalyptus has a strong aroma, but it can be helpful if your client is struggling with sinus issues or congestion. It also promotes sleep and relaxation and balances the Throat chakra.

- Neroli is a pleasant and relaxing floral scent that promotes restfulness and focus and helps balance the Crown and Heart chakras.

Music

I've been a musician for more than 40 years, so to me, music is as essential as breathing. In a Reiki session, music can hugely benefit you and your client. Playing appropriately relaxing music can help you focus, and it can relax your client. Additionally, music can act as a Reiki timer.

You'll find all kinds of Reiki timing music tracks anywhere you can download music, such as on YouTube and iTunes, and on smartphone apps. The music is usually quiet, soothing instrumental music that has a discreet chime or bell every three to five minutes that reminds you when it's time to change hand positions. This type of music is especially beneficial for first-degree Reiki practitioners who use the hand positions on themselves or others.

Music can also be an important part of the atmosphere of your Reiki sessions. Along with soft lighting, pleasant scents, a comfortable table, and a comfortable room temperature, music can help create a relaxing atmosphere that allows your clients to reach a receptive state as you channel Reiki energy to them.

Here are some things to consider with music:

- In general, it's best to avoid music with lyrics, as the words can be distracting.

- New age music is often a good choice because of its soothing cadence, melodies, and harmonies.

- Some classical music may also be a good choice, but avoid anything too stirring (no *1812 Overture* with cannon fire).

- Try to avoid music that has a familiar melody (usually elevator music is out for this reason); thinking of the lyrics or tracing the melody can be distracting.

- Search the term "Reiki timer music" on the Internet, and chances are you'll find something appropriate to help as you channel Reiki to your clients.

4 Healing Yourself

One of the benefits of Reiki is that you can channel the energy to yourself whenever you need it. As I mentioned, I recommend channeling Reiki to yourself every day at least for the first 21 days after any attunement, and then as often as needed. I generally channel Reiki to myself every day, even if only for a short time. You can channel Reiki to yourself during meditation (which is when I typically do it), or whenever you are sitting and not doing anything else with one or both of your hands, such as when you are watching television or reading a book.

Preparation

While you can channel Reiki to yourself casually, as when you are watching television or relaxing, I also recommend at least once a week (after the initial 21 days) channeling Reiki to yourself in a more formal manner, where you use prescribed hand positions for three to five minutes. While Reiki travels where it is needed regardless of how you channel it, giving yourself a formal Reiki session once a week serves as a sort of energetic tune-up, and it can help you reconnect to the Reiki energy in a profound manner.

When you perform such sessions, it's helpful to prepare your space to create the energetic environment and ambience to support healing and spiritual well-being.

PREPARING YOUR HEALING SPACE

I love my Reiki healing space I've set up in my home. It is in a quiet location away from my four dogs and one cat, and it is a space I have dedicated entirely to my Reiki, energy healing, meditation, and similar spiritual activities. It is a comfortable space with an energetic environment that supports a deeper dive into my connection with the divine. In the space, I've adjusted the lighting, created comfortable spots for meditation and Reiki, introduced aromatherapy, and placed objects I find sacred around the room. I also have a desk dedicated solely to my spiritual and energy healing writing and work.

For me, a majority of my second floor is dedicated to this space; I'm using my adult son's old loft-style bedroom. However, no matter how large or small your home is, it's important to carve out a space dedicated to your practice (or, if you plan to practice in an office, dedicate part of that space to Reiki). It doesn't have to be huge. It can be a corner of a room somewhere. Here are some important guidelines to setting up your practice space:

- Find a way to separate your practice space from other living spaces. So, if it's a room, make sure it has a door that closes. If it's a corner of a room, consider using divider screens or curtains to create separation.

- Ideally, your Reiki space should be away from areas of your home where you perform household tasks.

- Your space should limit visits from other people and pets as much as possible. If you can't always keep other people and pets out, consider a corner of a room with a door that closes, or put up a baby gate to keep others out when you use it.

- In your healing space, you may want a Reiki treatment table if you plan to channel the energy to others. You can buy a portable table that can be stored out of the way if you're using the space for something else or if it's a small space.

- For meditation, create an area in the corner with comfortable cushions. (I use a cushion specifically designed for meditation.)

- A well-ventilated area with soft or adjustable lighting is best.

- Consider placing sacred objects, such as crystals, statues, Himalayan salt lamps, and so on, around the area or on an altar in your dedicated space. In my space, I have various crystals, as well as two Himalayan salt lamps, and I burn candles in Himalayan salt candle holders.

- Consider scenting your space with relaxing aromas from candles, incense, or an aromatherapy diffuser. (I use an aromatherapy diffuser.)

- Use a speaker, such as the one on your device, to play music for relaxation and to use as your Reiki timer. (I use my laptop, although I do have a sound system in my space.)

Consider a ritual to cleanse and prepare your space before every session. For example, to prepare my space before a session, whether

Reiki for self-healing (self-Reiki) or performing Reiki on someone else, I burn chips of palo santo, a sacred wood, in the space, moving about the room and fanning the smoke in all corners in a counterclockwise direction. Then, I use tingsha (small cymbals) or a singing bowl for a minute or two. Finally, I channel Reiki into all four corners of the space by drawing CKR in each corner as well as across windows and doorways. You'll find your own ritual for preparing your space.

PREPARING YOURSELF

Next, you need to prepare yourself. Here are three suggested steps:

1. Dr. Usui recommended sitting in Gassho for about five minutes and gently focusing on the place where your middle fingers connect. This is typically how I recommend meditating before a session on yourself or anyone else, but you can meditate in any way that works for you.

2. After your meditation, silently or aloud, ask the Reiki to flow and ask to be guided in your Reiki session for the highest and greatest good. Mentally invite Reiki masters past and present, including Dr. Usui, Dr. Hayashi, and Madam Takata, to help you as you channel Reiki for the highest and greatest good.

3. When you feel ready, begin your session.

The Reiki Healing Technique

When you perform Reiki on yourself, you can use the 13 basic hand positions for self-healing (see page 54), or you can use a more intuitive approach. I use a combination of intuitive self-Reiki and hand positions. Most days of the week, I perform intuitive self-Reiki, but at least once a week (and more if I am sick or struggling emotionally or spiritually), I use all of the 13 hand positions. I also try to seek Reiki from other practitioners a few times a year just because I feel it's a good way to shake up the energy a bit and free energetic blockages I may not be finding on my own.

When you first start with self-Reiki, I recommend working with the 13 hand positions and playing a bit with intuitive Reiki to see how it works for you. So you might start with 5 to 10 minutes of intuitive Reiki followed by the 13 hand positions in each session. As you develop more intuitively, you might start to change this ratio, and eventually some of your sessions may be entirely intuitive. However, I do recommend performing all of the 13 hand positions at least once a week. I also recommend getting a Reiki treatment from someone else whenever possible. In my house that's pretty easy, because my husband is also a Reiki practitioner.

THE 13 BASIC HAND POSITIONS OF SELF-HEALING

The following are the 13 hand positions of self-healing with Reiki. You will use these hand positions daily for 21 days after any degree attunement, as well as whenever you channel Reiki to yourself. You can use the hand positions in order or follow your own intuitive guidance. Hold each for three to five minutes to channel Reiki. I like to do this in conjunction with meditation. You could also visualize the energy entering you through your hands and flowing to exactly where you need it to serve the highest and greatest good.

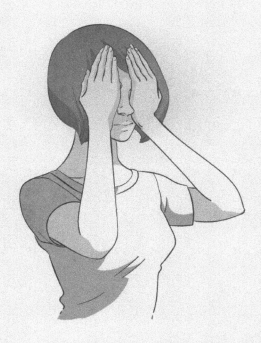

Eyes

Lightly cup both of your hands with your thumbs tucked along the side of each hand. Place the heels of your hands along either cheekbone, with your fingertips resting along your hairline above your forehead. Hands should only touch lightly on your cheekbones and hairline, and should be cupped over your eyes and brows without touching them.

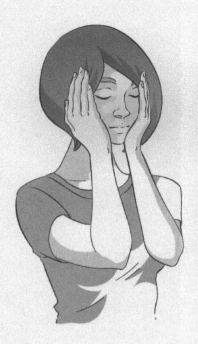

Cheeks

Cup both of your hands with the thumbs tucked along the side of each hand. Place your cupped hands over your cheeks, with your fingertips touching your temples along the side of your face and the heels of your hands lightly touching the sides of your jaw. To hold your hands in position, move your thumbs away from the side of the hands and hook them around the backs of your ears from the underside. Your hands should only be touching your head with the fingertips at your temples and heels of the hands along your lower jaw.

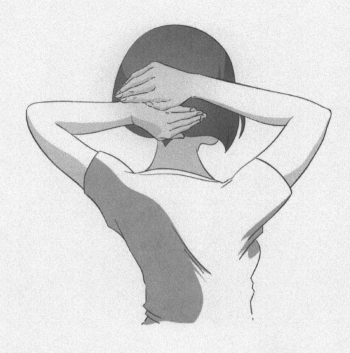

Back of Head

For this position, it doesn't matter which hand is on top; use whichever is most comfortable for you. Lightly cup your hands with your thumbs tucked along the side of each hand. Place your hands across the back of your head (fingertips pointing horizontally) with one hand stacked across your lower skull and one across the upper skull. Hands should be lightly cupped, with only the fingertips and heels of the hands touching along the sides of the back of your skull.

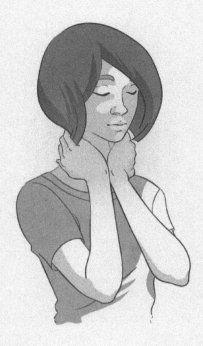

Side of Neck

Lightly cup your hands and rest them along the sides of your neck with your fingertips touching the back of your neck, the pinkie edge of your hand running along your lower jaw, and the heels of your hands resting along the front side of your neck with your thumbs tucked against the side of your hands along the collarbone.

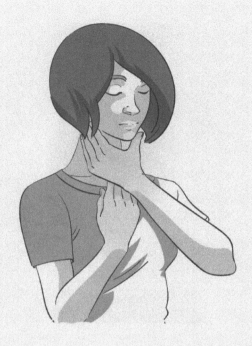

Throat and Heart

Place the fingertips of your left hand on your right jaw and the heel of your hand on your right upper chest so your hand is slanted slightly downward, keeping your hand cupped so only fingertips and heel touch your body. This allows this hand to cover your throat diagonally. With your right hand, rest your fingertips on the back of your left hand (or underneath the palm of your left hand), and rest the heel of your hand in the center of your chest.

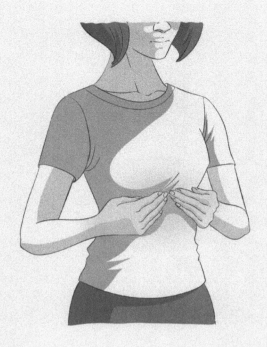

Ribs

Just under your breasts or chest, rest the fingertips of each hand along the bottom of your sternum with your fingertips together and your thumbs tucked alongside your hands. Cup your hands and extend your palms parallel to the floor with the pinkie side of your hands pointing downward and the heels of your hands touching along your rib cage on each side.

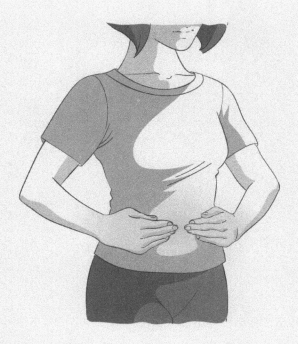

Abdomen

Place the middle finger of each hand on your belly button and hold each hand, fingers together, with your fingertips lightly touching the center of your abdominal region. Hold your hands with pinkie side parallel to the floor and extend your hands (lightly cupped) so the heels of your hands rest lightly along your sides.

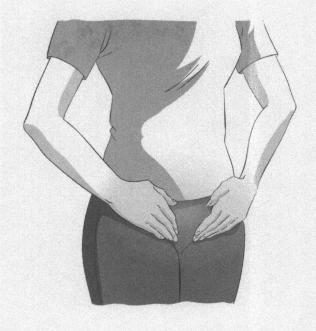

Groin

Place the heels of your hands along your outer groin where your legs meet your abdomen and you fold naturally to sit. Cup your hands, holding the thumbs tucked in, and place your fingertips along the inner thigh.

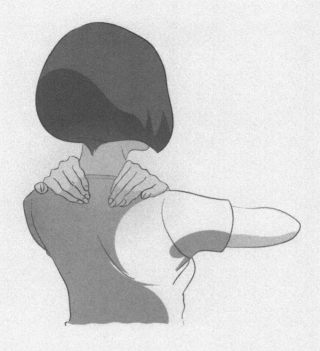

Shoulders

You can either cross your arms to do this or keep them uncrossed—whichever is most comfortable for you. For me, crossed works better. Place the fingertips of each hand along the top of the upper scapula along the back of your shoulder, and cup your hands over the top of the shoulder with the heels of your hands resting along the collarbone.

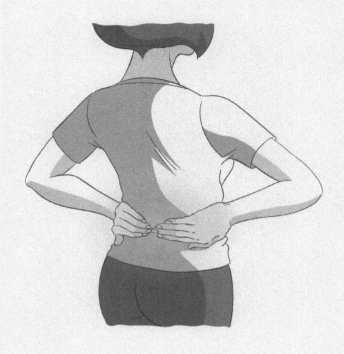

Middle Back

I like to think of this as the chicken-wing position, because your bent elbows extend from your body like chicken wings. Place the heel of each hand with your thumb side down along the sides of your rib cage, and curl your hands around the back so your fingertips rest on your latissimus dorsi (the muscles that run along the sides of your back), pointing toward your spine.

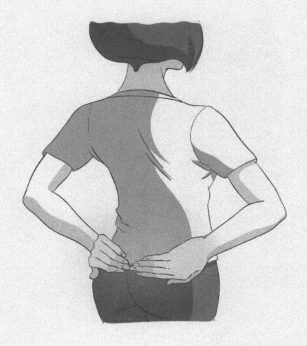

Lower Back

Place the heels of your hands along your sides just above your hips and curl your fingertips toward your spine so they rest in a line along the top of the rear of your pelvic bone.

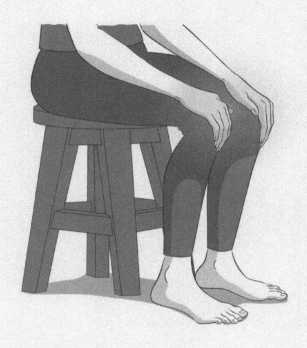

Knees

Cup your hands with your thumbs tucked along the side of each hand. Place the heels of your hands along the top of each knee and curve the fingers downward over the kneecap so the tips rest on your shinbones beneath the knees.

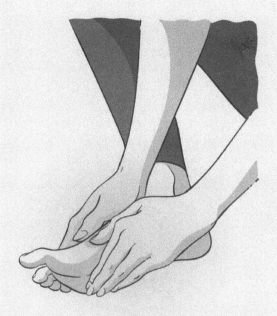

Feet

Working one foot at a time (so technically, it's 14 hand positions), cup the palm of one hand over the bottom of one foot and the other hand over the top.

REIKI TOUCH TECHNIQUES

Along with the hand positions, you can also use any of the following techniques as you feel is appropriate. While these are not typically taught as Reiki techniques, if you feel intuitively guided to do so, you may use them to direct or stimulate energy. These are all optional techniques, so use them only if you feel comfortable doing so and are intuitively guided to do so.

Touching
Touch lightly with your entire hand anywhere you feel you may need a little extra love.

Massaging
Using your palms and fingers, lightly massage areas of tension.

Tapping
There's a method called Emotional Freedom Technique (EFT) that involves tapping on various points firmly with the pads of the index and pointer fingers. If you feel guided to tap, you can use a firm tap with these two fingers for 8 to 10 taps, or as long as you are guided to do so. The Reiki prescriptions in chapters 6 and 7 occasionally tell you where to tap. Otherwise, listen to your intuition for location, or refer to techniques such as EFT to give you more information about tapping. If you are a second-degree practitioner or master-teacher, you can also visualize tapping the Reiki symbols into various points using this technique.

Stroking
Channeling Reiki through your palms, use long, smooth strokes if you feel guided to do so. This technique can soothe and also help direct energy.

Blowing
One of the techniques of Japanese Reiki is called Koki ho, and it involves blowing Reiki energy and symbols into various points. To do this, breathe Reiki in through your Crown chakra and visualize

Reiki symbols under the roof of your mouth while you silently intone the symbol name three times. Then, blow the Reiki into your hands and then apply it to yourself with the hands. You can also do this on others. Blow the Reiki from the roof of your mouth into the body, while visualizing the energy and symbol coming from you on your breath and going into the other person.

Gazing

Another Japanese Reiki technique called Gyoshi ho involves sending the loving life force of Reiki through the eyes. To do this, visualize Reiki flowing in through your Crown chakra and filling your head. When you are ready, gaze (without focusing) at the area on yourself where you'd like to direct the Reiki, and feel it flow through your eyes and into that part.

Distance Self-Healing

While it may seem like an oxymoron to send Reiki to yourself at a distance, I use this technique when I need some work on an area I can't reach very well or comfortably—for instance, pain in my scapula. It's tough to hold my hands there for long. So instead, I either visualize drawing the Reiki sandwich there and feeling the energy flow, or I use something as a surrogate for me (a stuffed animal, for instance), and using the Reiki symbols, I practice a distance healing session on myself.

A Full Reiki Self-Healing Session

When you perform a full Reiki self-healing session, you are your client. It's important to create just as sacred of a healing experience for yourself as you do for your clients. I realize sometimes it's more difficult to do this, and I fully admit to performing Reiki on the fly sometimes. (I've been known to channel Reiki whenever I find the time, such as when I'm riding in the car.) However, I do try to take time out of every day, even if it's only five minutes, to engage in the ritual of Reiki. For me, it is a meditative practice that helps keep me in an optimal spiritual, mental, and emotional space.

Create your environment. Just as you would with a client, create the optimal environment for healing. Set aside the time and space to do this where you are unlikely to be disturbed. Turn off your phone. If you're using your phone or computer for your music, disable any audio alerts and set your phone to airplane mode so you are not disturbed by random sounds.

Remove jewelry. This is an optional step, but it's one many Reiki masters and practitioners prefer. I actually choose to leave my jewelry on, because it is crystal jewelry programmed with certain intentions to facilitate healing. It's up to you what you decide to do here. Do what you are intuitively guided to do.

Sit comfortably. Whether in a chair, on the sofa, or on a cushion on the floor, sit comfortably. Rest your feet flat on the floor if you are in a chair to facilitate grounding, or sit in the lotus position (or another similar, comfortable position) if you are on the floor. Make sure your legs and feet are uncrossed (unless you're in the lotus position). Hold your spine erect with your shoulders comfortably back and sit back on your sit bones.

Spend five minutes meditating. Whether you use Gassho or something else, spend about five minutes clearing your mind, breathing deeply and comfortably into your belly. You can also use a mantra or affirmation here, such as "I am in optimum health," or a statement of intention such as, "I receive Reiki for my highest and greatest good."

Center yourself. After meditation, bring yourself back to center. Focus on your Hara (also known as the *dantian* or *dan t'ian*), which is the center of your prana or qi (life force energy). The Hara is about a hand's width below your navel. Place your hands here, resting them gently, and feel the warmth of prana building below them. If it helps, visualize the energy growing under your hands as a pink ball of light.

Ask the Reiki to flow. Put your hands together in Gassho and invite the Reiki to flow.

State your intention for the highest and greatest good. Once you feel the Reiki flow, invite Reiki masters past, present, and future to join you in channeling Reiki to serve your highest and greatest good. Set aside any preconceived notions or expectations as you do so, and simply allow the Reiki energy to do what is most needed.

Take a few minutes to practice intuitive Reiki. With your hands in Gassho, ask where the Reiki is most needed and wait for guidance. This may appear as a thought in your head, or you may notice a sensation in part of your body. Move your hands to this position and hold them there as long as you intuitively feel is necessary. Return to Gassho and ask again. Do this until you no longer feel guided or for a few positions before moving into the traditional hand positions.

Use the hand positions for a full self-Reiki session. Hold each hand position, in order, for three to five minutes. If you are guided by intuition to do so, perform other Reiki or touch techniques as you feel they are needed.

Return to Gassho and give thanks. At the end of the session, return to Gassho. Give thanks to Reiki, the universe, and Reiki masters past, present, and future, including Dr. Usui, Dr. Hayashi, and Madam Takata, for the healing that has occurred.

Ground yourself. Following your session, ground yourself by touching the floor with your hands, drinking a glass of cold water, or performing a simple grounding meditation such as visualizing roots growing from your feet into the center of the Earth.

Healing Others

CHAPTER 5

As you channel Reiki to others, it flows through you and they draw it in. One of the nice things about this is that as you treat others, you are also experiencing the Reiki energy working in you.

The great thing about starting with self-healing is you already have the basics in place for when you begin to work with others. You already know how to set up your environment and the things you need to make a session work. This is all quite helpful when you begin to work on healing others.

Be as Prepared as You Can Be

When I started channeling Reiki, I did so to a very skeptical husband—affectionately nicknamed Techie McScienceGeek because of his nuclear engineering training and his highly skeptical side-eye to anything not solidly grounded in strict scientific principles. With him, I didn't start with a full Reiki treatment. Instead, we focused on a persistent area of pain, his elbow, and I would sit snuggled up next to him on the couch channeling Reiki for 20 or 30 minutes to the pain he'd had there for several months.

After a few sessions, his pain disappeared permanently, and my skeptical hubby was ready to explore Reiki more fully. Unfortunately, all we had were beds, chairs, couches, and, sadly, no Reiki tables. Instead, I attempted to perform a full hands-on session using all of the hand positions by contorting myself into any number of uncomfortable positions around him. Knowing that wouldn't work for the long term, I invested in a Reiki table. It made everything easier.

Which is my way of telling you this: As soon as you think you can afford one, a Reiki or massage table is an essential investment. It creates a professional atmosphere, sets the stage, and makes it far more comfortable for you to perform hands-on Reiki sessions because you can move freely around your client and place your hands in appropriate positions. Also, if you are working with clients, you'll need a table to present an appropriate and professional treatment surface.

The preparation section in the previous chapter will help you as you begin to establish your own Reiki space for healing others. If you plan to do it professionally, having a separate and private space away from other areas of your home is essential. So is creating an atmosphere that is sacred and relaxing, to help make your clients comfortable and establish the right meditative mood for your own practice.

Techniques

As I mentioned in the previous chapter, all of the healing techniques described there can also be used on clients. You can use any of them—tapping, stroking, massage, blowing, gazing, and touching—with your clients, as long as they are comfortable with touch. I always begin every session by asking my clients if they are comfortable with me performing various techniques. If the answer is no (including touching), then I avoid those techniques.

If you have a client who is uncomfortable with touch, you can hold the Reiki hand positions an inch or two above their body. The Reiki will still channel effectively, and your client will be more comfortable with the session.

THE 12 BASIC HAND POSITIONS (AND 4 OPTIONAL HAND POSITIONS ALONG THE BACK)

There are 12 basic hand positions for a full Reiki session. Some Reiki master-teachers (including mine) teach an additional four positions along the back, which you can choose to incorporate as you wish. When performing a hands-on session, use a very light touch.

Have your client lie on their back on the table with their legs extended and arms at their sides. Ask them to uncross arms, legs, or feet, if they have them crossed.

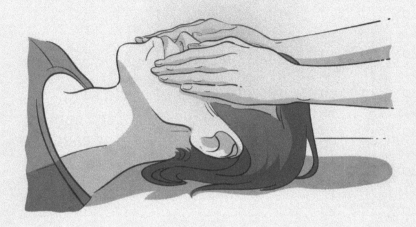

Eyes

Stand or sit at the crown of your client's head. Cup your hands lightly, with your thumbs tucked alongside the edge of each hand. Lightly rest your fingertips on your client's cheekbones, cup your hands over the eyes without touching them, and lightly rest the heels of your hands on the forehead.

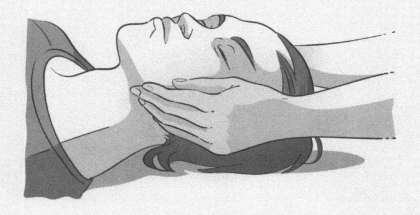

Ears

Still seated or standing at your client's crown, place the heels of your hands on your client's temples with your fingertips pointing down the length of their body. Lightly cup your hands with your thumbs tucked alongside each hand, and hook your pinkies lightly around your client's ears. Rest your fingertips along the jawline.

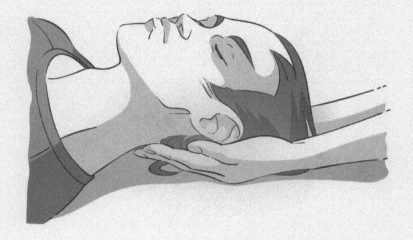

Back of Head

Still at your client's crown, place your hands under your client's head, taking the weight of their head in your hands. Place your fingertips along the occipital bone at the back of the skull and the heels of your hands along the back part of the top of their head. Cup your hands and tuck your thumbs in along the sides of your hands.

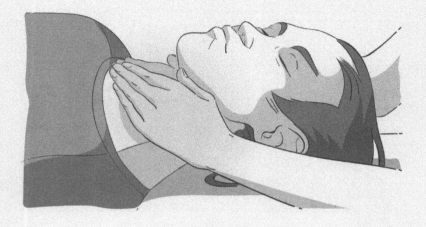

Throat

Remain at your client's crown. Be careful with this hand position that you don't place your hands directly across your client's throat, because it can make them feel uncomfortable and claustrophobic. Instead, place the heel of each hand along the collarbone where it meets the shoulder, and cup your hands with your thumbs tucked in along the sides of your hands. Place your fingertips along the top of the sternum so your hands run downward alongside the front of the throat.

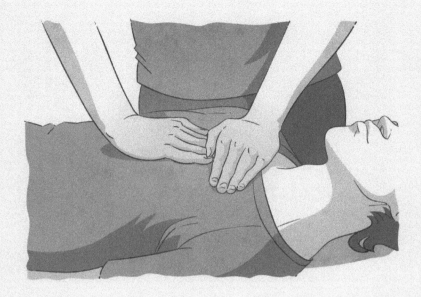

Heart

Move to either side of your client. Place the heel of one hand in the center of the chest along the sternum, resting the fingertips along the pectoral muscle above the breast, cupping your hand with your thumb tucked in along the side of your hand. Place the fingertips of your other hand along the back of your first hand with the heel resting along the sternum below the breasts. Be sure not to cup the breasts, which may make female clients uncomfortable.

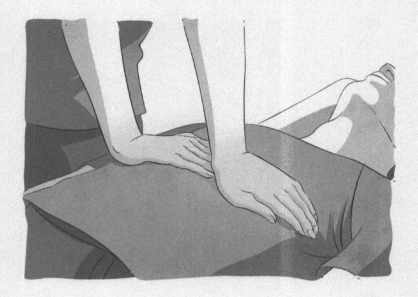

Solar Plexus

Still standing alongside your client, place the fingertips of which-ever hand is the most comfortable on the sternum below the breastbone, and place the heel on the rib cage with your hand cupped and your thumb tucked along the side of the hand. Place the heel of your other hand at the fingertips of your first hand and cup your hand, with your fingertips touching the opposite side of the rib cage.

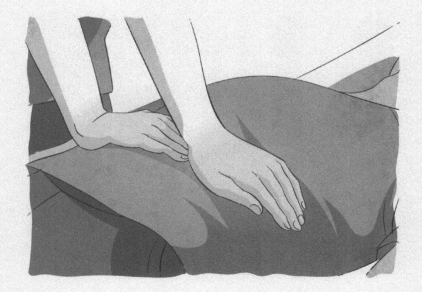

Navel

Standing at your client's side, place the fingertips of one hand (whichever is most comfortable) at the belly button and extend your hand so the heel touches along the obliques (the side abdominal muscles), keeping your hands cupped and your thumb tucked in along the side of your hand. Place the heel of your other hand along the fingertips of the first hand, and extend the fingertips to the other side of the obliques.

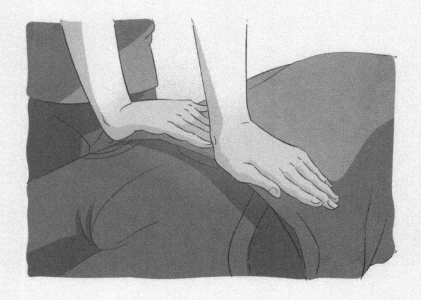

Hara

Perform the same hand position as Navel, one hand's width lower on the body.

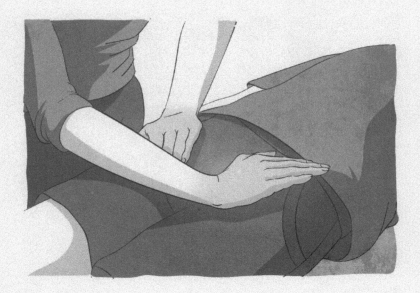

Groin

Still standing alongside your client, place the heel of whichever hand feels most comfortable at the crease of the outer hip along the top of the leg, with the fingers extending inward along the crease of the hip. Place the heel of the other hand near the inner crease of the hip and the fingertips near the outer crease.

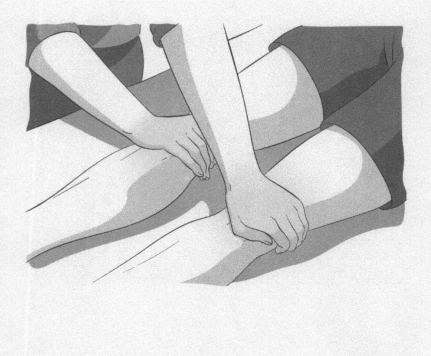

Knees

At your client's side, place one hand on each knee, with the heel of each hand on one side of the kneecap and the fingertips on the other side, so the palms are cupped over the knees.

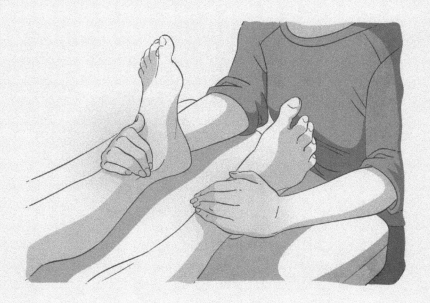

Ankles

At your client's side, place one hand along the front of each ankle with the heel of each hand on one side and the fingertips on the other, cupping your hands across the ankles.

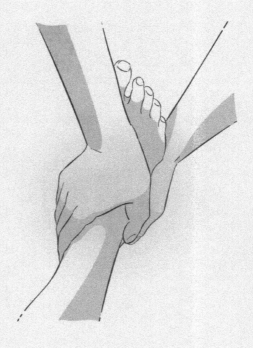

Feet

Stand at your client's feet, and work one foot at a time. Hold the arch of the foot in one hand and cup the top of the foot with your other hand.

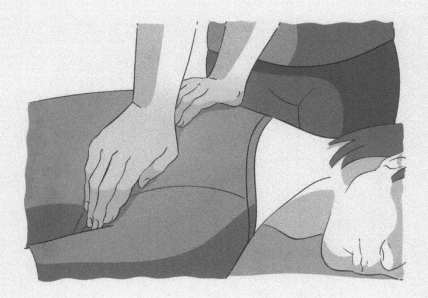

Shoulders

Standing at your client's side, place your hands in a line across the back of the shoulders with the fingertips of one hand and the heel of the other on the spine.

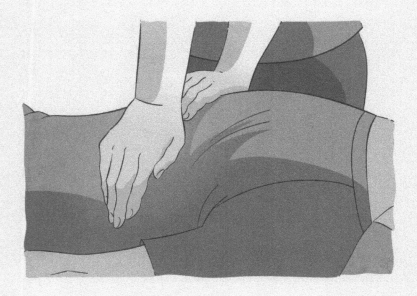

Middle Back

Standing at your client's side, place your hands in a line across the back at approximately the bra line (or the corresponding location on male clients) with the fingertips of one hand and the heel of the other on the spine.

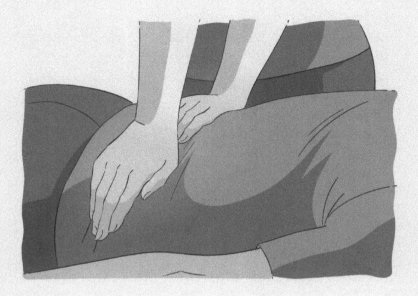

Lower Back

Standing at your client's side, place your hands in a line across the lower back, about waist level, with the fingertips of one hand and the heel of the other on the spine.

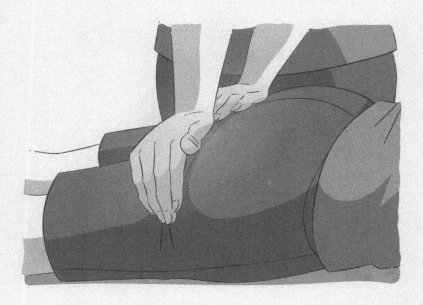

Tops of Legs

Standing at your client's side, place your hands in a line across the backs of the thighs, where the tops of the thighs meet the buttocks.

Preparing Your Subject

Along with preparing your own mindset via Gassho, meditation, inviting Reiki to flow, stating intention, and centering (as I described in the previous chapter on self-healing), you also need to prepare your client for the session, as follows:

Start with any intake paperwork. Have your client fill out any intake forms and sign an informed consent.

Ask if they have concerns or questions. Discuss them if so.

Ask if they are okay with touch or any other techniques you may use. If not, adjust as needed. As I mentioned earlier, you can hold the Reiki hand positions an inch or two above their body.

Explain to your client what to expect. Tell your client what will happen during the session. Explain that you will be holding various hand positions and channeling Reiki energy. Tell them you will channel the Reiki, and they will draw the Reiki in as you channel it. Tell them to relax, and explain that there is nothing they need to do except allow the experience. Explain that they may notice things such as warmth, swirling lights, visions, or emotional release, or they may experience nothing or even fall asleep. All are normal and occur as needed for their highest and greatest good.

Sweep your client's aura. Many Reiki practitioners start and end a session by sweeping the aura, the energy field that surrounds the body. (I encourage my students to do this.) Sweeping the aura can help clear any energetic imbalances from the aura, preparing your client for a full Reiki session. To sweep the aura, have your client stand in front of you. Holding your hands about three to five inches away from the body, start by cupping both hands over the top of their head without touching them. Now, sweep your hands in long, downward motions through their aura, working your way in long strokes down all planes of the body (front, sides, and back) through the auric field without touching the person. As you sweep, occasionally flick any energy from your hands by flicking your fingers downward toward the Earth and allowing the Earth to absorb any negative energy you've removed. Finish by sweeping from head to feet again and touching the ground to ground the energy.

Ask your client to relax and breathe as you prepare. Explain that you will prepare for a few minutes, and invite them to close their eyes and focus on their breathing as you complete your preparations to treat them. Suggest they release any expectations or preconceived notions as they relax and that they silently invite the Reiki energy to serve their highest and greatest good as you prepare. You may choose to meditate now if you haven't already done so to prepare for the session, depending on what seems appropriate for that particular client.

Performing a Session

When both you and your client are ready, you may perform your session. In general, sessions last about 30 minutes to an hour. You can perform an intuitive session, a session using all of the hand positions, or a combination of both.

PERFORMING A HANDS-ON SESSION

To perform a hands-on session, you will prepare as outlined earlier and then perform the 12 to 16 hand positions as outlined in the hand positions sections earlier in this chapter. Hold each position for three to five minutes.

ADRENALS HAND POSITION

Although the Adrenals hand position isn't one that is traditionally taught with Usui Reiki, I use it quite a bit in the prescriptions in chapters 6 and 7.

Your adrenal glands release your stress hormones. These stress hormones trigger the fight-or-flight response that was necessary to keep early humans from being killed and eaten by predators.

Today, we no longer need to fear being eaten by predators, but our adrenal glands don't know that. And so, when stress arises, they continue to release the hormones as if our lives depended on it. Unfortunately, we live in a chronically stressful environment. The pressures of daily life, our jobs, world events, and many other factors keep our adrenals in a constant state of hormone production and release. The result is that they can become chronically exhausted, which can lead to a host of other mental, emotional, and physical problems. Therefore, I find channeling Reiki directly to the adrenals in many of the prescriptions to be helpful for exhausted glands, and I offer the Adrenals hand position as part of many remedies.

To channel Reiki to the adrenals, place the heel of each hand on the rib cage just below the breasts/chest, with the fingers of each hand pointed toward the sternum. Hold the position for three to five minutes, as you would any other hand position. You can make this part of your regular rotation of hand positions, or use it just for specific remedies, knowing Reiki always flows to where it is needed most.

PERFORMING AN INTUITIVE SESSION

To perform an intuitive session, in your preparation, ask that you channel the Reiki to serve the highest and greatest good of your client. Then do the following:

1. Stand at either the crown of your client's head or at their feet with your hands in Gassho and ask to be guided.

2. When you receive guidance, move to that position and hold the hand position there. Hold it for three to five minutes, or until you are guided to move.

3. Return to the head or feet, stand with your hands in Gassho again, and ask for guidance to the next area.

4. Do this until you are no longer guided, or until the time you have set aside for your session has expired.

5. If you receive no guidance, simply do the hand positions as you would a hands-on session.

REIKI BOX

You can use a Reiki box to channel Reiki to several people at once. To do this, write their names on a piece of paper (or use pictures of them). Place them in a box together. Prepare as you always do, and then draw the Reiki sandwich on your hands, saying the name of each symbol three times as you draw it to activate it. Channel Reiki to the box until you feel the session is complete. You can also write the names of situations or world events and put them in the Reiki box to send Reiki energy.

ENDING A SESSION

At the end of each session, do the following:

1. When the session ends, stand with your hands in Gassho at your client's crown or feet and give thanks to Reiki, Dr. Usui, Dr. Hayashi, Madam Takata, and your client for allowing you to channel the Reiki (you can do this silently or aloud).

2. Then, silently state your intention for your client to go forward in health and wellness toward their highest and greatest good.

3. Gently tell your client to sit up on the table when they are ready.

4. Sweep their aura while they are in a seated position.

5. Give them a drink of cold water to ground them after the session.

6. Run your hands under cold water to break the energetic link between the two of you and to ground yourself.

7. Spend additional time with your client as needed. Suggest they drink plenty of plain water throughout the day to flush out any toxins released during their session, and tell them to allow any emotions that may arise in the wake of the session. Remind them that you are available if they have questions and let them know how to contact you.

QUICK SESSION HAND POSITIONS

If you don't have a full hour for a session, you can perform a quick session with nine hand positions held for two to three minutes each. Have your client sit on a chair with their feet flat on the floor and their arms at their sides. Then complete the hand positions on the following pages:

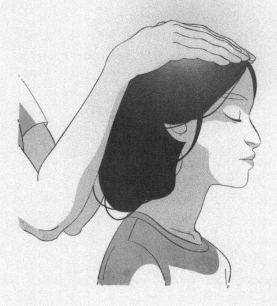

Crown Chakra

Standing behind your client, cup your hands over the top of the head with your fingertips resting on the forehead and the heels of your hands resting lightly on the back of the skull.

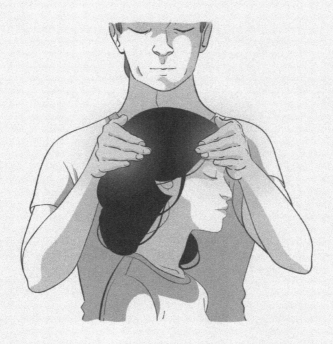

Third Eye Chakra

Standing to one side of your client, cup your hands and place one in front of your client's forehead with your fingertips and the heel of your hand resting on either side of the forehead and the fingertips and heel of your other hand resting along each side of the back of the head.

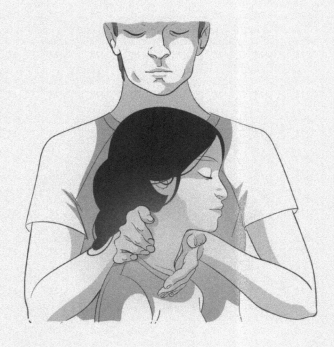

Throat Chakra

Standing to one side of your client, cup your hands in front of the throat and in back of the neck, with the fingertips and heels of your hands resting lightly on each side of the neck.

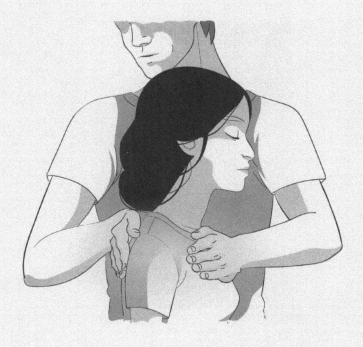

Heart Chakra

Standing to one side of your client, place the heel of your forward hand in the center of the sternum with the fingertips angled up and resting above the breast. Cup your back hand above the spine at heart height with the fingertips and the heel of your hand resting on each side of the spine.

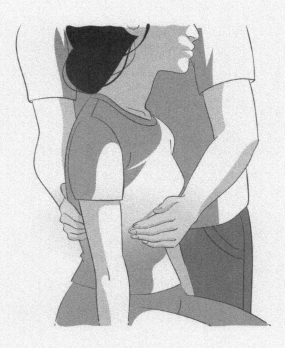

Solar Plexus Chakra

Standing to one side of your client, cup your forward hand over the base of the sternum with your fingertips and the heel of your hand resting on each side of the sternum. Place your back hand at the same height cupped across the spine, with the fingertips and heel resting on each side of the spine.

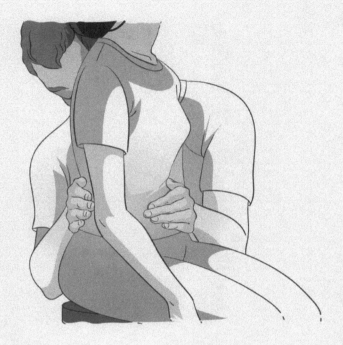

Sacral Chakra

Standing to one side of your client, cup your hands across the midline of your client's abdomen on one side and their spine at the same level on the back, one hand's width beneath the belly button at Hara level.

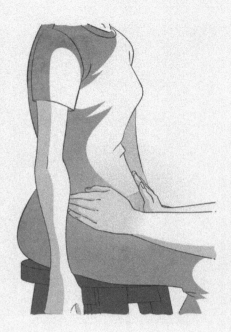

Root Chakra

Stand or kneel in front of your client. Place one hand across each leg where their leg folds into the sitting position.

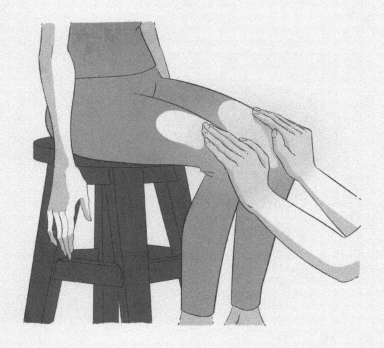

Knees

Kneeling or sitting in front of your client, cup one hand over each of their knees.

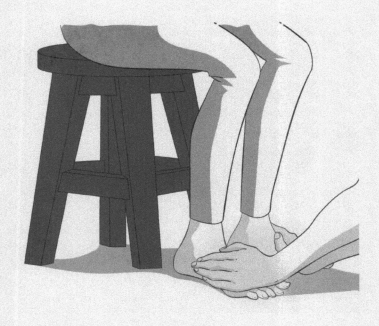

Feet

Kneeling or sitting in front of your client, cup one hand over the top of each of their feet.

Distance Healing

Once you are attuned to second-degree Reiki, you can send Reiki healing at a distance using the Reiki sandwich (CKR + SHK + CKR + HSZN + CKR) to channel Reiki energy across space and time. There are several distance healing techniques you can use.

SURROGATE TECHNIQUE

With the surrogate technique, you can use a stuffed animal or a doll as a stand-in for your Reiki client. To perform the technique, follow these steps:

1. Set a time with your client. At that time, ask your client to sit comfortably and quietly for 30 to 60 minutes (or for however long you schedule your Reiki session).

2. About five minutes before your Reiki session, prepare yourself, meditate, sit in Gassho, and ask the Reiki to flow. Then hold your surrogate object and indicate that the Reiki is intended for your client (state your client's name aloud or silently and try to visualize your client), and the object will serve as a surrogate.

3. Draw the Reiki sandwich on each of your hands, intoning the name of each symbol three times.

4. Perform a hands-on Reiki session using the surrogate, just as you would if your client were there. Using a doll in this way, your hand positions will be much closer together. If your hands cover more than one of the traditional positions, then you don't need to do both. Just move on to the next position after the three to five minutes.

5. When you are done, give thanks to Reiki and your client, and run your hands under cold water to break the energetic connection between you.

MINI ME TECHNIQUE

In this technique, you can use a small object as a stand-in for your client. I like to use a crystal, a photograph, or a piece of paper with the client's name written on it. This channels Reiki to your client's whole being at one time, so it is much faster than using the surrogate method.

1. Set a date and time with your client and ask them to sit quietly for about 20 minutes at the given time.

2. About five minutes before your set time, begin your preparations with meditation and Gassho.

3. Draw the Reiki sandwich on both of your hands, making sure you say the name of each symbol three times as you draw it to activate the symbols.

4. State the intention that the paper, image, or whatever you are using as your stand-in will serve as the surrogate for your client.

5. When you feel the Reiki begin to flow, hold the surrogate between your hands and channel Reiki to it for about 5 or 10 minutes, or until you feel the session is complete.

6. Give thanks to Reiki and your client, and run your hands under cold water to break the energetic connection between you.

Healing Children

Working on children is similar to working on adults. All of the techniques and hand positions are the same. However, it is important to always have a parent present when you channel Reiki to a child. You may also want to shorten sessions with children, or if the child or parent is uncomfortable with hands-on healing, use the technique where your hands are a few inches above your subject.

DISTANCE HEALING ETHICS

There are a few ethical issues associated with distance healing that are important to keep in mind:

- Never channel Reiki to someone else at a distance without securing their permission.
- If it's an emergency and you are unable to get permission, you can channel Reiki to that person but intend that if the person doesn't want to receive the Reiki, it goes where it serves the highest and greatest good.
- If you've set up a time and date with someone to channel Reiki, make sure you do as you've said you would. It's never okay to tell someone you will channel Reiki to them and then not do so.
- When you send Reiki across time or distance to an event, such as after a natural disaster, intend that it go where it is most needed to serve the highest and greatest good.

- For very young children, distance healing techniques or very short sessions are best. Children have small bodies, and the Reiki doesn't have as far to flow, so if you do a hands-on session, you may want to work with a short intuitive session as opposed to a full 12-hand-position session; use only three or four hand positions lasting only two or three minutes each. If the child seems uncomfortable at all, stop and try again another time.
- Always make sure you have the parent or guardian's consent before working with a child, whether in person or at a distance. You'll need the same paperwork and documentation for a child as you would for an adult.

- Always be sensitive in working with children to avoid touching any private areas (any place a bathing suit might cover). In these areas, hold your hands two to three inches above them instead of directly touching the area.

- Take cues from the child you're working on. If they start to get wiggly, they may be uncomfortable, or they may feel done with the session. Ask if they'd like you to stop, and follow the child's direction so you don't overtire them. The goal is to give them small amounts of Reiki and have them find it a pleasant experience so it is something they continue to seek as they get older. Forcing a child to lie still for a 60-minute session is likely too much, so always keep their attention span in mind when working with kids.

- Another technique you can use with children is to have their parents place their hands in a hand position directly on the child, and then you place your hands over the parent's hands and channel the Reiki through them. For shy children, this may be a better option.

- You can also use distance Reiki techniques to send Reiki to a child who is a few feet away, if touch seems inappropriate for the situation. Distance healing may also be appropriate with children who seem uncomfortable with hands-on healing.

Healing Pets

I have four small dogs and a cat, and they have different reactions to Reiki. My 14-year-old toy fox terrier, Spike, likes Reiki and lies still for it. I suspect the warmth feels good in his old bones. My dogs Mickey and Sofie usually don't want anything to do with Reiki or will only tolerate it for a short period. They may sit still for a minute or two of hands-on Reiki, but then they're off and doing their own thing. My cat can take or leave Reiki, so we may try short sessions here and there. My five-pound Brussels griffon, Monkey, however, has never seen a Reiki session she didn't want to be involved in. She's always working her way under my hands, especially if she sees me channeling Reiki to one of the other dogs or to my husband when she's in the room. She loves Reiki and never seems to tire of it.

I quickly came to recognize how each of my pets responded to Reiki based on their reactions to it, and I work within what they indicate they will tolerate. All of my pets are under 15 pounds, so they are very light and have small bodies. When I channel Reiki to them, I do it in short increments—about 5 to 10 minutes max, as part of petting or cuddle sessions. The exception is Monkey. When she's in my lap and my hands aren't doing anything else, I'm channeling Reiki to her. Sometimes when my hands are doing something else, she still works her way under them, demanding Reiki.

Pay attention to the cues your pets give you. Start with channeling Reiki for a minute or two during cuddle time and see how they respond. You'll be able to tell quite quickly and can adapt your strategy from there. Typically, your sessions with your pets will be much shorter and intuitive. I find that pets all sort of wiggle around to get my hands where they feel they need the Reiki the most. I allow them to guide the session, instead of insisting on anything formal. For larger pets, such as horses or large dogs, you may want to approximate the human hand positions on them, taking care to ensure you maintain your own safety as you work with them. If, at any time, they seem uncomfortable, stop.

For pets who aren't snugglers—or pets you probably shouldn't touch, like fish—you can also use distance Reiki. You can do this using a surrogate or the mini me technique and channeling Reiki for about five minutes.

I also channel Reiki to my pets when I am away from home. I use a distance Reiki method (usually mini me or the Reiki box) and channel Reiki to each of them several times throughout the day. I believe this helps them remain calmer and feel more connected to me when I am away from home for extended periods. Even if I can only do this for a minute or two at a time, it helps me stay connected to them, especially Monkey, who tends to have separation anxiety when I'm gone.

When working with your pets, use your intuition and let them lead the way. They will let you know by their actions what they need and respond to best. Start with short sessions and try for longer periods as the pet seems willing, but don't force it.

Healing Plants and Food

Rumor has it around my house that I am a plant serial killer. Or I used to be. I was never great with plants, and it took me many years to realize I somehow killed even the hardiest of plants, regardless of what I believed were my best efforts to keep them alive. But then I started Reiki, and a few years later, I got up the courage to try my hand at plants again. They're not dead yet.

You can use Reiki for your plants. I do, and it seems to be correcting any deficiencies in my ability to care for them and keep them alive. Here are a few methods you can use with plants:

- Place your hands around the container that holds the plant and channel Reiki to the roots for about five minutes once or twice a week (or when intuitively guided to do so).

- Channel Reiki energy to the food and water you provide your plants. This is my main method. I hold the watering can with the water in it and channel Reiki for about five minutes, and then water the plants. So far, so good.

- Channel Reiki to seeds before you plant them.
- Channel Reiki to the soil before planting seeds or transplanting stems.

I'm also a big believer in channeling Reiki to food and drink. We have so many foods and beverages in our diet that don't support optimal health, and I believe channeling Reiki to the food before we eat it can help set the intention that the food and drink nourish us as we need. To channel Reiki to food and beverages, try any of the following:

- Hold your hands an inch or two above your plate of food and channel Reiki for one to two minutes.
- Hold food in your hands (such as an apple or pear) and channel Reiki to it.
- Channel Reiki to the water you use to water vegetables or fruits you grow.
- Hold a beverage in a glass and channel Reiki to it for two minutes.
- If you are a second-degree practitioner, draw the CKR symbol over food or beverages before you consume them.
- If you are a master-teacher, draw the DKM symbol over food or beverages before you consume them.

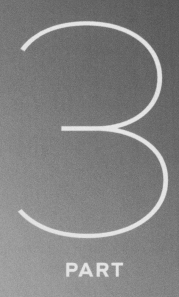

PART

Healing 100+ Ailments

6

Physical Healing

Reiki is an intelligent energy: It goes where it's needed, regardless of where you place your hands. Likewise, when you do use the hand positions, you direct Reiki evenly throughout the body. However, in some cases, your clients will come to you with a specific diagnosis from a physician or a health problem they are experiencing. When they do, you can also supply directed energy as a complementary treatment to their primary care from their physician. Using directed treatments may save time in a Reiki session, or it may allow you to focus more on specific problems.

Things to Consider Before Doing Directed Treatment

While your Reiki treatment can complement treatment from a primary health-care provider, it's important to consider the following before using Reiki to work with a specific health condition.

- Unless you are a medical doctor or have some other degree or training that allows you to diagnose patients (such as physician's assistant, chiropractor, naturopath, or nurse practitioner), you must never diagnose a client. You are prohibited from doing so both legally and ethically.

- The treatments listed in this chapter are not intended to diagnose any condition, nor are they suggested as a replacement for primary health care from licensed professionals. Rather, they are intended as complementary treatment and should be presented as such to your client. Never tell a client they should stop therapy prescribed by their health-care providers.

- Unless you have other certifications (such as LMT, registered dietician, etc.), limit your treatment to only Reiki and other energy modalities (such as crystals). Do not prescribe diet, herbal remedies, or other modalities of treatment unless you have a license to do so.

- Many health-care facilities, such as hospitals and nursing homes, may prohibit any modalities other than those offered by people employed by or contracted with that facility. Therefore, before offering Reiki in a medical facility of any kind, check with the facility administration to ensure your hands-on care is allowed in the facility.

- Never contradict a diagnosis or treatment recommendation from licensed health-care professionals.

- If possible, when seeing clients for specific health conditions, try to have a referral from a medical doctor.

- It's important to let your clients know you cannot guarantee any results and that Reiki healing occurs in the highest and greatest good of the client. It's important both you and your client release any expectations or requirements for how the Reiki energy may bring about healing.

Channeling Reiki for Specific Body Parts

With the previous guidelines in mind, if a client complains of issues in a certain area of the body, along with recommending they seek medical evaluation, diagnosis, and treatment from the appropriate health-care professional, you can try certain Reiki techniques to help improve energy flow in the affected area. For all hand positions (see chapter 5) except sweeping the aura, hold the position for three to five minutes. Begin and end each sequence by sweeping your client's aura.

Channeling Reiki for Specific Ailments

If your client has been diagnosed with a specific ailment by a medical professional, use the following treatments to supplement appropriate health care. Never diagnose these problems yourself, never suggest a physician's diagnosis is incorrect, and never suggest your client stop their medical treatments or pursue only alternative modalities. Your role in treating these ailments is to offer Reiki as a complement to appropriate medical care.

Abdomen

Chakra: Sacral

Abdominal issues may be something as simple as a stomachache or a pulled abdominal muscle, or may be a more complex health issue.

* Hara, Navel, and Lower Back (with client lying facedown) hand positions balance Sacral chakra

SEQUENCE

1. *Touch:* Hara
2. *Touch:* Navel
3. *Touch:* Lower Back (with client lying facedown)

OTHER TECHNIQUES

Place a piece of carnelian on your client's Hara.

Allergies

Chakra: Heart

Allergies are an immune system response to certain substances in food or airborne particles. They have varying degrees of severity and may be associated with the adrenal glands. They can affect the lungs, throat, and sinuses.

- Eyes and Ears hand positions balance sinuses, Eustachian tubes, and lymph glands
- Throat hand position balances throat
- Heart hand position balances lungs and Heart chakra
- Solar Plexus hand position balances adrenal glands
- Adrenals hand position balances adrenal glands

SEQUENCE

1. *Touch:* Eyes
2. *Tap:* Two-finger tap along sinuses in counterclockwise direction
3. *Touch:* Ears
4. *Stroke:* Stroke palms from backs of ears along sides of neck to shoulders
5. *Touch:* Throat
6. *Touch:* Heart
7. *Touch:* Solar Plexus
8. *Touch:* Adrenals

OTHER TECHNIQUES

After step two in the sequence, place small pieces of rainbow fluorite along the lower sinuses.

Anemia

Chakra: Crown, Third Eye, Heart

Many things cause anemia, including hemorrhage, lifestyle choices, and congenital factors. It is primarily a circulation issue (Heart chakra), but if it is associated with bleeding, it is also a Third Eye chakra issue. Bone marrow builds blood, so balancing the Crown chakra (which supports the skeletal system) can help.

- Eyes and Ears hand positions balance Crown and Third Eye chakras
- Heart hand position balances circulatory system and Heart chakra
- Solar Plexus hand position balances adrenal glands

SEQUENCE

1. *Touch:* Eyes
2. *Touch:* Ears
3. *Touch:* Heart
4. *Touch:* Solar Plexus

OTHER TECHNIQUES

Bloodstone and hematite help increase blood volume. Place a piece of either stone under the treatment table.

Ankles

Chakra: Root

Ankle issues may arise as the result of many conditions, such as lower back issues or misalignments of the angles of the quadriceps.

- Groin hand position balances Root chakra
- Knees hand position balances legs
- Ankles hand position works both ankles to balance energy

SEQUENCE

1. *Touch:* Groin
2. *Stroke:* Stroke palms down upper thigh to top of knee
3. *Touch:* Knees
4. *Stroke:* Stroke palms from knee to ankle
5. *Touch:* Ankles (cup hands around each side of ankle)

OTHER TECHNIQUES

Place a piece of red garnet on the treatment table between your client's ankles.

Arthritis

Chakra: Sacral

Work arthritis from two angles: channel Reiki energy to the Sacral chakra, which is associated with arthritis, and then work on the affected areas.

- Navel and Hara hand positions balance Sacral chakra

SEQUENCE

1. *Touch:* Navel
2. *Touch:* Hara
3. *Touch:* Any areas of pain, stiffness, and inflammation (hold hand positions over areas of pain, using a light touch)

OTHER TECHNIQUES

Baltic amber fights inflammation. Recommend that your client wear it on or near areas of pain and inflammation.

Asthma

Chakra: Heart

Asthma originates in the Heart chakra and affects the sinuses, throat, and ears. If your client is experiencing an active asthma attack, which can be life-threatening, they must seek emergency medical treatment before pursuing relief from energy healing.

- Eyes and Ears hand positions support sinuses
- Throat hand position supports throat
- Heart and Middle Back (with client lying facedown) hand positions balance Heart chakra
- Adrenals hand position supports adrenal glands, which asthma medications affect

SEQUENCE

1. *Touch:* Eyes
2. *Tap:* Two-finger tap around sinuses counterclockwise
3. *Touch:* Ears
4. *Stroke:* Stroke palms from the backs of ears along sides of neck to shoulders
5. *Touch:* Throat
6. *Touch:* Heart
7. *Touch:* Adrenals
8. *Touch:* Middle Back (with client lying facedown)

OTHER TECHNIQUES

Have your client lie on their back with eyes closed, breathing deeply, and visualize a green healing light entering through the nose, traveling through the nasal passages into the lungs, and expanding to fill all parts of lungs with healing light. As the client exhales, they visualize completely exhaling any toxins. They can do this at home and during the treatment for as long as they would like.

Autoimmune Conditions

Chakra: All

According to the American Autoimmune Related Diseases Association, there are more than 100 autoimmune diseases, and they can affect all parts of the body. Autoimmune conditions occur when the immune system sees the body's own tissue as a foreign invader and attacks it. While you'll also want to use Reiki to balance energy related to the symptoms of the various autoimmune conditions, balancing the chakras can help the whole body function optimally.

- Eyes, Ears, and Throat hand positions balance Crown, Third Eye, and Throat chakras
- Heart hand position balances Heart chakra
- Solar Plexus hand position balances Solar Plexus chakra
- Hara hand position balances Sacral chakra
- Groin hand position balances Root chakra

SEQUENCE

1. *Touch:* Eyes
2. *Touch:* Ears
3. *Touch:* Throat
4. *Touch:* Heart
5. *Touch:* Solar Plexus
6. *Touch:* Hara
7. *Touch:* Groin

OTHER TECHNIQUES

Run a chakra-balancing line of crystals along the floor under the treatment table, as follows:

- Root: hematite
- Sacral: carnelian
- Solar Plexus: citrine
- Heart: rose quartz
- Throat: chalcedony
- Third Eye: amethyst
- Crown: clear quartz

Bronchitis

Chakra: Heart, Throat

Bronchitis is an inflammation in the bronchial tubes that causes bronchial spasms and coughing. It may occur in the wake of a cold or the flu, or it may be chronic. To work with a client with bronchitis, supporting the Heart chakra is helpful, as is providing support to sinuses and throat.

- Eyes and Ears hand positions balance sinuses and Eustachian tubes
- Throat hand position balances Throat chakra
- Heart and Middle Back (with client lying facedown) hand positions balance lungs and Heart chakra
- Ribs hand position alleviates rib pain from coughing

SEQUENCE

1. *Touch:* Eyes
2. *Touch:* Ears
3. *Touch:* Throat
4. *Touch:* Heart
5. *Stroke:* Stroke palms in counterclockwise circles on upper chest
6. *Touch:* Ribs (palms lightly on ribs under breasts, with fingers extended toward sternum)
7. *Stroke:* With client lying facedown, stroke palms in counterclockwise circles along scapula on both sides of spine
8. *Touch:* Middle Back (with client lying facedown)

OTHER TECHNIQUES

Recommend your client wear a Baltic amber necklace or bracelet to help fight lung inflammation.

Circulation

Chakra: Heart

Circulation problems are associated with the Heart chakra, although they may also be associated with the specific area where circulation is an issue. Because some circulation problems can be life-threatening, it's essential to have your client seek medical attention before working with energy healing.

- Heart hand position balances Heart chakra and supports circulation
- Touching areas where circulation is an issue stimulates circulation in that area

SEQUENCE

1. *Touch:* Heart
2. *Stroke:* For poor circulation in the extremities, stroke palms in long, gentle strokes along affected extremities
3. *Touch:* Any area where circulation is an issue

OTHER TECHNIQUES

In the palm of your hand, add one drop of ginger essential oil to one tablespoon of sweet almond oil. Warm it between your hands and use it to gently stroke areas of impaired circulation.

Colds and Flu

Chakra: Root, Throat

Colds and flu are caused by an external virus, but some people are especially susceptible to them because of impaired immunity. Therefore, along with treating areas affected by cold or flu, balance the Root chakra energy to enhance immunity. Since adrenal exhaustion can also lead to decreased immunity (or result from illness), balancing the adrenal glands is necessary as well. Balancing the Throat Chakra is important since colds and flus so often affect the throat.

- Eyes and Ears hand positions balance sinuses and Eustachian tubes
- Throat hand position balances Throat chakra
- Heart hand position helps chest congestion
- Adrenals hand position supports adrenal glands
- Groin hand position balances Root chakra

SEQUENCE

1. *Touch:* Eyes
2. *Tap:* Two-finger tap along brows
3. *Tap:* Two-finger tap along cheekbones
4. *Touch:* Ears
5. *Touch:* Throat
6. *Touch:* Heart
7. *Touch:* Adrenals
8. *Touch:* Groin

OTHER TECHNIQUES

Diffuse orange and cinnamon essential oils during the session to boost immunity.

Constipation

Chakra: Root

Energy blockages in the Root chakra cause constipation, which may also be associated with issues in the spine above the problem, so working with spinal points in the neck and middle back may also be helpful.

- Throat hand position for neck support
- Heart hand position for upper back support
- Solar Plexus hand position for middle-back support
- Hara hand position for intestinal support
- Groin hand position balances Root chakra

SEQUENCE

1. *Touch:* Throat
2. *Touch:* Heart
3. *Touch:* Solar Plexus
4. *Touch:* Hara
5. *Touch:* Groin

OTHER TECHNIQUES

Place a piece of red garnet on the treatment table between your client's legs.

Crohn's Disease, Colitis, Irritable Bowel Syndrome

Chakra: Root

All three illnesses listed here are intestinal autoimmune conditions. Therefore, the Root chakra comes into play, since it supports immunity and is also associated with conditions of the intestines and bowel.

- Hara and Lower Back (with client lying facedown) hand positions for intestinal support
- Groin and Tops of Legs (with client lying facedown) hand positions balance Root chakra

SEQUENCE

1. *Touch:* Hara
2. *Touch:* Groin
3. *Touch:* Lower Back (with client lying facedown)
4. *Touch:* Tops of Legs (with client lying facedown)

OTHER TECHNIQUES

If you are a second-degree Reiki practitioner, draw CKR on the lower back to strengthen immunity.

Diabetes

Chakra: Solar Plexus, Root

Diabetes is a pancreas (Solar Plexus chakra) and hormonal disorder. Type 1 diabetes is an autoimmune condition (Root chakra), while type 2 diabetes is a metabolic disorder. At this time, research hasn't been able to completely classify type 2 diabetes as an autoimmune condition, but it doesn't hurt to treat it energetically as if it is.

- Solar Plexus and Middle Back (with client lying facedown) hand positions balance Solar Plexus chakra and pancreas and provide metabolic support
- Groin hand position balances Root chakra

SEQUENCE

1. *Touch:* Solar Plexus
2. *Touch:* Groin
3. *Touch:* Middle Back (with client lying facedown)

OTHER TECHNIQUES

Place a piece of citrine under the treatment table.

Diarrhea

Chakra: Root

Diarrhea comes from overactive energy associated with the Root chakra and intestines. Recommend medical evaluation if your client has had diarrhea for more than a few days, if they are in a high-risk population (such as very young, elderly, or immunocompromised), or if they are showing signs of dehydration. Like constipation, diarrhea can originate farther up the spine.

- Throat hand position balances neck
- Heart hand position balances upper back
- Solar Plexus hand position balances middle back
- Hara and Lower Back (with client lying facedown) hand positions balance intestines
- Groin and Tops of Legs (with client lying facedown) hand positions balance Root chakra

SEQUENCE

1. *Touch:* Throat
2. *Touch:* Heart
3. *Touch:* Solar Plexus
4. *Touch:* Hara
5. *Touch:* Groin
6. *Touch:* Lower Back (with client lying facedown)
7. *Touch:* Tops of Legs (with client lying facedown)

OTHER TECHNIQUES

Place a piece of hematite on the treatment table between your client's legs.

Ears

Chakra: Third Eye, Throat

Issues of the ear, such as ear pain, tinnitus (ringing in the ears), vertigo, and congestion, may result from an imbalance between the Third Eye and Throat chakras.

- Eyes hand position balances Third Eye chakra and sinuses
- Ears hand position balances ears
- Throat hand position balances ears, Eustachian tubes, and Throat chakra

SEQUENCE

1. *Touch:* Eyes
2. *Tap:* Two-finger tap brow bone from inner brow outward to temples
3. *Tap:* Two-finger tap cheekbones
4. *Touch:* Ears
5. *Stroke:* Stroke palms downward along the jawline, ending at chin
6. *Touch:* Throat

OTHER TECHNIQUES

Diffuse eucalyptus essential oil during the session.

Eating Disorders

Chakra: Solar Plexus, Root

Eating disorders have both a mental and a physical basis. They are associated with the Solar Plexus chakra, but the addictive elements of these conditions often originate in the Root chakra. If your client is dealing with an eating disorder, recommend medical and mental health evaluations.

- Throat hand position helps dental issues and throat problems associated with some eating disorders
- Solar Plexus and Middle Back (with client lying facedown) hand positions balance adrenals and Solar Plexus chakra
- Adrenals hand position balances adrenal glands
- Groin, Lower Back (with client lying facedown), and Tops of Legs (with client lying facedown) hand positions balance Root chakra

SEQUENCE

1. *Touch:* Throat
2. *Touch:* Solar Plexus
3. *Touch:* Adrenals
4. *Touch:* Groin
5. *Touch:* Middle Back (with client lying facedown)
6. *Touch:* Lower Back (with client lying facedown)
7. *Touch:* Tops of Legs (with client lying facedown)

OTHER TECHNIQUES

Recommend your client repeat daily affirmations such as, "I am optimally healthy and strong, and I choose nutritious foods that support my well-being."

Elbows

Chakra: Heart, Throat, Crown

Elbow issues may result from overuse or may be related to systemic issues, such as arthritis, or energetic issues of the associated chakra (Heart chakra). Neck problems (Throat chakra) may also cause elbow pain, or the pain may be skeletal (Crown chakra).

- Eyes and Back of Head hand positions balance Crown chakra
- Throat hand position balances Throat chakra
- Heart hand position balances Heart chakra
- Elbow hand position works both elbows to balance energy

SEQUENCE

1. *Touch:* Eyes
2. *Touch:* Back of Head
3. *Touch:* Throat
4. *Touch:* Heart
5. *Stroke:* Stroke palms from shoulders to elbows along sides of arms
6. *Touch:* Elbow (hands cupped on each side of the elbow)
7. *Stroke:* Stroke palms from elbows to wrists along forearms

OTHER TECHNIQUES

In the palm of your hand, add one drop of frankincense essential oil to one teaspoon of sweet almond oil. Rub the oil between your palms and use as you stroke from elbows to wrists.

Eyes

Chakra: Third Eye

Eye issues include pain, blurred vision, fatigue, or more serious diagnoses.

- Eyes, Ears, and Back of Head hand positions balance Third Eye chakra, eyes, and facial nerves

SEQUENCE

1. *Touch:* Eyes
2. *Touch:* Ears
3. *Touch:* Back of Head
4. *Touch:* Eyes

OTHER TECHNIQUES

Place a piece of amethyst under the treatment table at the level of the Third Eye chakra.

Fatigue

Chakra: Solar Plexus, Crown, Third Eye

Many things cause fatigue, such as hormonal disorders or poor-quality sleep (Third Eye chakra), adrenal issues (Solar Plexus chakra), or lifestyle choices. Crown chakra imbalances can cause fatigue. Therefore, balancing the crown can help.

- Eyes, Ears, and Back of Head hand positions balance Crown and Third Eye chakras
- Adrenals hand position balances adrenal glands
- Solar Plexus hand position balances Solar Plexus chakra and adrenals

SEQUENCE

1. *Touch:* Eyes
2. *Tap:* Two-finger tap along cheekbones
3. *Touch:* Ears
4. *Touch:* Back of Head
5. *Tap:* Two-finger tap along collarbone on each side of sternum
6. *Touch:* Adrenals
7. *Tap:* Two-finger tap on Heart chakra
8. *Touch:* Solar Plexus

OTHER TECHNIQUES

Diffuse orange, lemon, or grapefruit essential oils, or a combination of them, during the session.

Feet

Chakra: Root

Foot problems may originate in the feet or anywhere above them, such as the ankles, knees, hips, or lower back.

- Groin hand position balances Root chakra
- Knees hand position balances leg energy
- Ankles hand position balances ankle energy
- Feet hand position provides energy and balance to feet

SEQUENCE

1. *Touch:* Groin
2. *Stroke:* Stroke palms from tops of thighs to knees
3. *Touch:* Knees
4. *Stroke:* Stroke palms from base of knees down shins to ankles
5. *Touch:* Ankles
6. *Touch:* Feet (use two hands for each foot)

OTHER TECHNIQUES

Place a piece of hematite on the treatment table between your client's feet.

Fibroids

Chakra: Sacral

Fibroids are benign tumors that grow in the uterine walls. Some are asymptomatic, but others cause pain, pressure, and heavy menstruation. Working with fibroids is a matter of balancing energy in the Sacral chakra.

- Navel, Hara, and Lower Back (with client lying facedown) hand positions provide Sacral chakra and uterine support

SEQUENCE

1. *Touch:* Navel
2. *Touch:* Hara
3. *Touch:* Lower Back (with client lying facedown)

OTHER TECHNIQUES

Recommend your client wear an amber ring or bracelet for support.

Head

Chakra: Crown, Third Eye, Throat

General issues of the head, such as mind fog, headaches, or congestion, are common and are related to the Crown and Third Eye chakras. Neck issues (Throat chakra) may also contribute.

- Eyes, Ears, and Back of Head hand positions balance Crown and Third Eye chakras
- Throat hand position balances Throat chakra

SEQUENCE

1. *Touch:* Eyes
2. *Touch:* Ears
3. *Sweep:* Sweep palms lightly from ears along jawbone to chin
4. *Touch:* Back of Head
5. *Touch:* Throat

OTHER TECHNIQUES

Diffuse grapefruit essential oil during the session.

Headache, Migraine

Chakra: Crown, Third Eye

Headaches originate in the Third Eye and Crown chakras. However, tension headaches may arise from tension in the neck or jaw (Throat chakra), while migraines may be related to circulation (Heart chakra). Sinus headaches may also be a problem.

- Eyes, Ears, and Back of Head hand positions balance Crown and Third Eye chakras
- Throat hand position balances Throat chakra
- Heart hand position balances Heart chakra

SEQUENCE

1. *Touch:* Eyes
2. *Touch:* Ears
3. *Touch:* Back of Head
4. *Touch:* Throat
5. *Touch:* Heart

OTHER TECHNIQUES

Place a piece of amethyst on the treatment table near your client's head.

Heart

Chakra: Heart

Never ignore heart issues or treat them lightly. Before you work on someone complaining of heart problems, it is essential they seek appropriate medical care. Only provide treatment after they've had a thorough medical evaluation and treatment. Never provide Reiki to someone who has a pacemaker, because Reiki energy may interfere with the pacemaker.

- Heart hand position balances Heart chakra
- Solar Plexus hand position balances Solar Plexus chakra
- Throat hand position balances Throat chakra

SEQUENCE

1. *Touch:* Heart
2. *Touch:* Solar Plexus
3. *Touch:* Throat
4. *Touch:* Heart

OTHER TECHNIQUES

Place a piece of rose quartz under the treatment table at the level of the heart.

Hemorrhoids

Chakra: Root

Inflammation in the rectal region (Root chakra) causes hemorrhoids. Straining, as with constipation, may also contribute, so if this is the case, you may also want to offer the constipation treatment.

- Groin and Tops of Legs (with client lying facedown) hand positions balance Root chakra

SEQUENCE

1. *Touch:* Groin
2. *Touch:* Tops of Legs (with client lying facedown)
3. *If constipation is an issue, continue with the guidelines on page 127.*

OTHER TECHNIQUES

Place a piece of red jasper on the treatment table between your client's legs.

Hips

Chakra: Sacral, Root

A Sacral chakra imbalance causes hip issues. Lower spine problems (Root chakra) may contribute. The other area of concern for hip problems are the knees and the angle of the hips in relation to the knees (known as the Q angle).

- Hara hand position balances Sacral chakra
- Groin hand position balances Root chakra
- Knees hand position balances knees
- Hips hand position works hips

SEQUENCE

1. *Touch:* Hara
2. *Touch:* Groin
3. *Stroke:* Stroke palms on each hip in a circular motion to release congestion
4. *Touch:* Hips (one hand on the outer portion of each hip)
5. *Stroke:* Stroke palms from upper thighs to knees along front of thighs
6. *Stroke:* Stroke palms along sides of thighs from hips to outer knees
7. *Touch:* Knees

OTHER TECHNIQUES

Diffuse patchouli essential oil during the session.

Inflammation

Chakra: Primarily Crown, All

Inflammation helps your body fight disease, but many people experience it in an unhealthy way, and it then causes chronic conditions, widespread pain, and illness. Imbalances of the Crown chakra can often result in systemic illnesses.

- Eyes and Back of Head hand positions balance Crown and Third Eye chakras
- Throat hand position balances Throat chakra
- Heart hand position balances Heart chakra
- Solar Plexus hand position balances Solar Plexus chakra
- Hara hand position balances Sacral chakra
- Groin hand position balances Root chakra

SEQUENCE

1. *Touch:* Eyes
2. *Touch:* Back of Head
3. *Touch:* Throat
4. *Touch:* Heart
5. *Touch:* Solar Plexus
6. *Touch:* Hara
7. *Touch:* Groin
8. *Touch:* For specific areas of inflammation, hold hands over inflamed areas

OTHER TECHNIQUES

Place four pieces of Baltic amber on the floor around the treatment table at your client's head, feet, and right and left hips.

Intestines

Chakra: Root

Intestinal issues are associated with the Root chakra.

- Groin hand position balances Root chakra
- Hara, Navel, and Lower Back (with client lying facedown) hand positions balance energy of upper intestines
- Tops of Legs (with client lying facedown) hand position balances lower intestines

SEQUENCE

1. *Touch:* Navel
2. *Touch:* Hara
3. *Touch:* Groin
4. *Touch:* Lower Back (with client lying facedown)
5. *Touch:* Tops of Legs (with client lying facedown)

OTHER TECHNIQUES

Place a piece of smoky quartz on the treatment table between your client's legs below the Root chakra.

Jaw, Mouth

Chakra: Throat

Jaw and mouth issues may include dental problems or pain, halitosis, or jaw pain. These are related to the Throat chakra.

- Throat hand position balances Throat chakra and neck and jaw energy
- Ears hand position balances jaw and mouth

SEQUENCE

1. *Touch:* Throat
2. *Tap:* Two-finger tap along jawbone from front of ears to chin on each side of face
3. *Touch:* Ears

OTHER TECHNIQUES

Diffuse clove essential oil, which is associated with the jaw and mouth, during the session.

Knees

Chakra: Root

Knee issues may originate in the joint itself or may be caused by something above it, particularly the lower back. They may also be affected by the Q angle between the hips and the knees.

- Groin hand position balances Root chakra
- Hips hand position balances hip energy
- Knees hand position balances knees
- Ankles hand position improves support to knees

SEQUENCE

1. *Touch:* Groin
2. *Touch:* Hips (hands on each side of outer part of hips)
3. *Stroke:* Stroke palms downward from tops of thighs to tops of knees
4. *Stroke:* Stroke palms from outer part of hips along sides of legs to sides of knees
5. *Touch:* Knees
6. *Touch:* Ankles
7. *Touch:* Knees

OTHER TECHNIQUES

Place a piece of black tourmaline on the treatment table between your client's knees.

Lower Back

Chakra: Root, Sacral, Crown, Third Eye

Lower back pain often has a severe effect on quality of life. Lower back problems originate in the Root or Sacral chakra but can also be related to poor posture (Root chakra), skeletal problems (Crown chakra), or spinal problems (Third Eye chakra). Knee, hip, and ankle issues may also cause lower back pain.

- Eyes and Back of Head hand positions balance Crown and Third Eye chakras and skeleton
- Navel and Hara hand positions balance Sacral chakra
- Groin and Lower Back (with client lying facedown) hand positions balance Root chakra
- Hips hand position balances hip energy
- Knees hand position balances knees
- Ankles hand position balances ankles
- Feet hand position grounds

SEQUENCE

1. *Touch:* Back of Head
2. *Touch:* Eyes
3. *Touch:* Navel
4. *Touch:* Hara
5. *Touch:* Groin
6. *Touch:* Hips (hands on each side of the outer part of the hips)
7. *Touch:* Knees
8. *Touch:* Ankles
9. *Touch:* Feet
10. *Touch:* Lower Back (with client lying facedown)

OTHER TECHNIQUES

Place a snowflake obsidian crystal under the treatment table at the mid-body level to help balance spinal energies.

Lungs

Chakra: Heart

With lung problems (Heart chakra), it's best to err on the side of caution and make sure your client gets an appropriate medical diagnosis and care before seeking alternative energy healing, as some lung issues can be serious or life-threatening.

- Heart hand position balances Heart chakra
- Solar Plexus hand position moves energy around Heart chakra
- Throat hand position moves energy around Heart chakra

SEQUENCE

1. *Touch:* Heart
2. *Touch:* Throat
3. *Touch:* Solar Plexus
4. *Touch:* Heart

OTHER TECHNIQUES

- Place a piece of moss agate under the treatment table.
- Use visualization meditation with your client during or after the session. Have them lie on their back, breathing deeply and imagining pulling healing energy in through their nose and into their lungs. As they exhale, have them visualize releasing through the breath any energies that don't serve them.

Menopause Problems

Chakra: Sacral

As women near menopause, the body's hormonal balance changes. Some women sail through menopause, and others struggle with moderate to severe symptoms. The severity of menopause is closely related to energy imbalances in the Sacral chakra. Because these issues can lead to adrenal exhaustion, the Solar Plexus chakra and adrenals are a secondary focus.

- Solar Plexus and Adrenals hand positions balance Solar Plexus chakra and adrenals
- Navel, Hara, and Lower Back (with client lying facedown) hand positions balance Sacral chakra

SEQUENCE

1. *Touch:* Solar Plexus
2. *Touch:* Adrenals
3. *Touch:* Navel
4. *Touch:* Hara
5. *Touch:* Lower Back (with client lying facedown)

OTHER TECHNIQUES

With you or on their own, encourage your client to chant the Bija mantra associated with the Sacral chakra: VAM (pronounced *vahm*). (Bija are special mantras that have the power to create transformative energy.)

Middle Back

Chakra: Heart, Solar Plexus, Third Eye, Sacral, Root, Crown

Middle-back issues may relate to Heart, Solar Plexus, or Sacral chakras. They may also arise from posture issues (Root chakra), spinal problems (Third Eye chakra), or issues of the skeletal system (Crown chakra).

- Eyes, Ears, and Back of Head hand positions balance Crown and Third Eye chakras
- Heart and Middle Back (with client lying facedown) hand positions balance Heart chakra
- Solar Plexus hand position balances Solar Plexus chakra
- Navel and Hara hand positions balance Sacral chakra
- Groin hand position balances Root chakra

SEQUENCE

1. *Touch:* Eyes
2. *Touch:* Ears
3. *Touch:* Throat
4. *Touch:* Back of Head
5. *Touch:* Heart
6. *Touch:* Solar Plexus
7. *Touch:* Navel
8. *Touch:* Hara
9. *Touch:* Groin
10. *Stroke:* With client lying facedown, stroke palms lightly downward from backs of shoulders to middle back along trapezius muscles
11. *Touch:* Middle Back (with client lying facedown)

OTHER TECHNIQUES

Sound a singing bowl, chime, or tuning fork tuned to F or F sharp before, during, or after treatment.

Neck

Chakra: Throat, Crown, Root, Third Eye

Neck problems originate in the Throat chakra. However, other issues may contribute, such as poor posture (Root chakra), spinal issues (Third Eye chakra), or musculoskeletal problems (Crown chakra). Shoulder tension may also contribute.

- Eyes, Ears, and Back of Head hand positions balance Crown and Third Eye chakras
- Throat and Shoulders (with client lying facedown) hand positions support neck and shoulders and balance Throat chakra

SEQUENCE

1. *Touch:* Eyes
2. *Touch:* Ears
3. *Touch:* Back of Head
4. *Stroke:* Stroke palms lightly along collarbone from shoulders to sternum
5. *Touch:* Throat
6. *Stroke:* With client lying facedown, stroke palms along backs of shoulders
7. *Touch:* Shoulders (with client lying facedown)

OTHER TECHNIQUES

- Place blue crystals on the treatment table on each side of your client's neck.
- With you or on their own, encourage your client to release neck tension by vocalizing the Bija mantra HAM (pronounced *hahm*). (Bija are special mantras that have the power to create transformative energy.)

PMS, Menstrual Pain

Chakra: Sacral, All

PMS and menstrual pain originate in the Sacral chakra and are primarily related to hormonal changes. However, exhaustion and mood issues, which are also related to PMS, may originate in the Crown and Root chakras. Hormonal issues may also take a toll on the adrenal glands, and adrenal exhaustion may contribute to menstrual disorders, as may thyroid issues.

- Eyes hand position balances Third Eye and Crown chakras
- Throat hand position provides thyroid support
- Heart hand position balances upper and lower chakras
- Solar Plexus and Adrenals hand positions provide adrenal support
- Navel and Hara hand positions balance Sacral chakra
- Groin hand position balances Root chakra

SEQUENCE

1. *Touch:* Eyes
2. *Touch:* Throat
3. *Touch:* Heart
4. *Touch:* Solar Plexus
5. *Touch:* Adrenals
6. *Touch:* Navel
7. *Touch:* Hara
8. *Touch:* Groin

OTHER TECHNIQUES

Create a chakra-balancing grid of crystals on the floor under the treatment table, as follows:

- Root chakra: hematite
- Sacral chakra: carnelian
- Solar Plexus chakra: Baltic amber
- Heart chakra: ruby in fuchsite
- Throat chakra: aquamarine
- Third eye chakra: lepidolite
- Crown chakra: howlite

Ribs

Chakra: Heart, Crown, Root, Third Eye

Rib issues are associated with the Heart chakra but may also relate to musculoskeletal (Crown chakra), spinal (Third Eye chakra), or posture (Root chakra) problems.

- Eyes, Ears, and Back of Head hand positions balance Crown and Third Eye chakras
- Heart and Middle Back (with client lying facedown) hand positions balance rib cage and Heart chakra
- Groin hand position balances Root chakra

SEQUENCE

1. *Touch:* Eyes
2. *Touch:* Ears
3. *Touch:* Back of Head
4. *Touch:* Heart
5. *Touch:* Groin
6. *Touch:* Middle Back (with client lying facedown)

OTHER TECHNIQUES

Have your client practice belly breathing. Lying on their back with eyes closed, your client breathes deeply into the belly, feeling it expand and visualizing the rib cage expanding with each inhale. Your client holds the breath for three seconds before exhaling completely. They can do this at home for 5 to 10 minutes or for as long as desired.

Sciatica

Chakra: Root

Sciatica occurs when a nerve (Third Eye chakra) in the lower back is pinched, shooting pain down the leg and into the foot. The Root chakra is the primary focus for sciatica, but working on the legs is important as well.

- Eyes hand position balances Third Eye chakra
- Hara and Lower Back (with client lying facedown) hand positions support lower back
- Groin and Tops of Legs (with client lying facedown) hand positions balance Root chakra
- Knees hand position supports legs
- Ankles hand position supports ankles
- Feet hand position supports feet

SEQUENCE

1. *Touch:* Eyes
2. *Touch:* Hara
3. *Touch:* Groin
4. *Stroke:* Stroke palms from tops of thighs to tops of knees
5. *Touch:* Knees
6. *Touch:* Ankles
7. *Stroke:* Stroke palms downward from knees to ankles
8. *Touch:* Feet
9. *Touch:* Lower Back (with client lying facedown)
10. *Touch:* Tops of Legs (with client lying facedown)

OTHER TECHNIQUES

Place a piece of rainbow fluorite on your client's Third Eye chakra.

Sexually Transmitted Infections

Chakra: Sacral, Root

Energy healing supports the immune system (Root chakra) as it fights sexually transmitted infections (STIs), and it may also alleviate symptoms. For STIs, focus on the sex organs (Sacral chakra) as well.

- Navel, Hara, and Lower Back (with client lying facedown) hand positions balance Sacral chakra
- Groin and Tops of Legs (with client lying facedown) hand positions boost immunity and balance Root chakra

SEQUENCE

1. *Touch:* Navel
2. *Touch:* Hara
3. *Touch:* Groin
4. *Touch:* Lower Back (with client lying facedown)
5. *Touch:* Tops of Legs (with client lying facedown)

OTHER TECHNIQUES

Place a piece of carnelian under the treatment table even with your client's Hara.

Shoulders

Chakra: Heart, Throat, Crown, Third Eye, Root

Shoulder problems are associated with the Heart chakra. However, neck (Throat chakra), musculoskeletal (Crown chakra), spinal (Third Eye chakra), and posture (Root chakra) issues may contribute.

- Eyes, Ears, and Back of Head hand positions balance Crown and Third Eye chakras

- Throat hand position balances neck and Throat chakra

- Heart and Shoulders (with client lying facedown) hand positions balance shoulders and Heart chakra

- Groin hand position balances Root chakra

SEQUENCE

1. *Touch:* Eyes

2. *Touch:* Ears

3. *Touch:* Back of Head

4. *Touch:* Heart

5. *Stroke:* Stroke palms from backs of ears along sides of neck to shoulders

6. *Touch:* Throat

7. *Touch:* Groin

8. *Stroke:* With client lying facedown, stroke palms from base of neck along spine outward along backs of shoulders

9. *Touch:* Shoulders (with client lying facedown)

OTHER TECHNIQUES

Breathing and visualization release shoulder tension. Your client sits, feet flat on the floor with eyes closed, breathing deeply into their belly through the nose. They visualize air pulling healing energy into the shoulder area, while lifting the shoulders to their ears. Then the client breathes out through the mouth, lowering the shoulders and visualizing tension leaving them. They can do this at home for 5 to 10 minutes or for as long as desired.

Sinus Congestion and Pain

Chakra: Third Eye, Throat

Sinus pain and congestion is related to imbalances in the Third Eye chakra, and it may also affect the throat and lungs.

- Eyes, Ears, and Back of Head hand positions balance Third Eye chakra
- Throat hand position supports throat and balances Throat chakra
- Heart hand position supports lungs

SEQUENCE

1. *Touch:* Eyes
2. *Touch:* Ears
3. *Touch:* Back of Head
4. *Touch:* Throat
5. *Touch:* Heart

OTHER TECHNIQUES

Sound a tuning fork, singing bowl, or chime tuned to A or A sharp before or after treatment.

Anytime your client experiences sinus pressure, they can use the following technique for a minute or two: Have the client "rock" their sinuses by placing their thumb on the bridge of the nose between the eyes and placing the tongue along the roof of their mouth behind the teeth, and firmly alternating pressing with thumb and tongue; this is an acupressure trick that really works to help clear the sinuses.

Sinuses

Chakra: Third Eye

Sinus problems, such as congestion, inflammation, and pain, are all related to the Third Eye chakra.

• Eyes and Ears hand positions balance Third Eye chakra

SEQUENCE

1. *Touch:* Eyes
2. *Tap:* Two-finger tap from each side of nose near bridge, moving downward along cheekbones to ears
3. *Stroke:* Stroke two fingers along brows, moving from nose outward to temples
4. *Stroke:* Stroke two fingers along cheekbones, moving outward to corners of eyes
5. *Touch:* Ears

OTHER TECHNIQUES

Diffuse two drops of eucalyptus oil, two drops of peppermint oil, and two drops of thyme oil during the session.

Stomachache, Nausea, Gastroenteritis

Chakra: Solar Plexus, Sacral, Root

Stomach problems occur in the abdomen, intestines, or near the diaphragm if acid reflux is an issue. Therefore, working with the first three chakras can help strengthen the entire system.

- Solar Plexus hand position balances Solar Plexus chakra and upper GI tract
- Navel hand position supports stomach and upper intestines
- Hara and Lower Back (with client lying facedown) hand positions balance Sacral chakra and support abdomen
- Groin and Tops of Legs (with client lying facedown) hand positions balance Root chakra and support lower intestines

SEQUENCE

1. *Touch:* Solar Plexus
2. *Touch:* Navel
3. *Touch:* Hara
4. *Touch:* Groin
5. *Touch:* Lower Back (with client lying facedown)
6. *Touch:* Tops of Legs (with client lying facedown)

OTHER TECHNIQUES

Diffuse ginger essential oil during the session.

Throat

Chakra: Throat

Throat problems arise from the Throat chakra and may include persistent sore throat, congestion, coughing, or laryngitis.

- Throat and Shoulders (with client lying facedown) hand positions balance Throat chakra
- Ears hand position balances upper throat and jaw

SEQUENCE

1. *Touch:* Ears
2. *Stroke:* Stroke palms from backs of ears along sides of neck to shoulders
3. *Touch:* Throat
4. *Touch:* Shoulders (with client lying facedown)

OTHER TECHNIQUES

During meditation at home, your client can try the following: Lying on their back, the client visualizes the throat as a swirling wheel of blue energy. They visualize white energy coming through the Crown chakra down through the Throat chakra and each remaining chakra, and exiting into the center of the Earth. You can also suggest they do this visualization during their treatment.

Thyroid Disorders

Chakra: Throat

The thyroid is the butterfly-shaped gland in the front of the throat that controls metabolism. Thyroid disorders may be autoimmune, so along with focusing on the Throat chakra, focus on the Root chakra to boost the immune system. Adrenal insufficiencies often go hand in hand with thyroid disorders, so focusing on adrenal support is essential as well.

- Throat hand position balances thyroid and Throat chakra
- Adrenals and Solar Plexus hand positions support adrenals
- Groin hand position supports immunity

SEQUENCE

1. *Touch:* Throat
2. *Touch:* Adrenals
3. *Touch:* Solar Plexus
4. *Touch:* Groin

OTHER TECHNIQUES

Sound a tuning fork, singing bowl, or chime tuned to G or G sharp before or after treatment.

Toothache

Chakra: Throat

The Throat chakra is energetically linked to the mouth. Therefore, when a client has dental problems, focus on the mouth, jaw, and throat region. For severe tooth pain, recommend a dental visit as soon as possible.

- Ears and Back of Head hand positions support jaw and mouth
- Throat hand position balances Throat chakra

SEQUENCE

1. *Touch:* Ears
2. *Touch:* Back of Head
3. *Touch:* Throat

OTHER TECHNIQUES

Diffuse clove essential oil during the session.

Urinary Tract Infection

Chakra: Sacral, Solar Plexus

Urinary tract infections (UTIs) present with pain, burning, and frequent urination. For some, they are chronic and occur regularly. The Solar Plexus chakra supports the energy of the kidneys and the Sacral chakra supports the energy of the rest of the urinary tract. Increasing immunity through the Root chakra can also help.

- Solar Plexus and Middle Back (with client lying facedown) hand positions balance kidneys and Solar Plexus chakra
- Navel, Hara, and Lower Back (with client lying facedown) hand positions balance Sacral chakra and support urinary tract
- Groin and Tops of Legs (with client lying facedown) hand positions boost immunity and balance Root chakra

SEQUENCE

1. *Touch:* Solar Plexus
2. *Touch:* Navel
3. *Touch:* Hara
4. *Touch:* Groin
5. *Touch:* Middle Back (with client lying facedown)
6. *Touch:* Lower Back (with client lying facedown)
7. *Touch:* Tops of Legs (with client lying facedown)

OTHER TECHNIQUES

Place pieces of deep-brown or orange Baltic amber on each side of your client's waist on the treatment table.

Varicose Veins

Chakra: Root, Heart

Varicose veins, which are enlarged and tangled veins, are most common in the legs and feet. They may not cause symptoms, or they may be painful, especially when standing and walking. The Root chakra controls the energy to the legs and feet, while the Heart chakra is associated with the circulatory system and blood vessels.

- Heart hand position supports circulatory system and blood vessels and balances the Heart chakra
- Groin hand position balances Root chakra
- Knees and Ankles hand positions support legs
- Feet hand position supports feet

SEQUENCE

1. *Touch:* Heart
2. *Touch:* Groin
3. *Touch:* Knees
4. *Touch:* Ankles
5. *Touch:* Feet

OTHER TECHNIQUES

With you or on their own, encourage your client to chant the Bija mantra LAM (pronounced *lahm*). (Bija are special mantras that have the power to create transformative energy.)

Vertigo

Chakra: Crown, Third Eye

Vertigo is connected to the Crown and Third Eye chakras. It may also be associated with the inner ears. Clients with vertigo should seek medical evaluation to make sure its cause is benign before seeking energetic solutions.

- Eyes and Back of Head hand positions balance Crown and Third Eye chakras
- Ears hand position supports inner ears
- Adrenals hand position (palms on the ribs just below the breasts with fingers pointed toward the sternum) helps vertigo related to exhaustion
- Feet hand position supports grounding

SEQUENCE

1. *Touch:* Eyes
2. *Touch:* Ears
3. *Touch:* Back of Head
4. *Touch:* Adrenals
5. *Touch:* Feet

OTHER TECHNIQUES

Suggest that anytime your client feels dizzy, they sit with their feet flat on the floor and visualize roots growing from their feet into the Earth for a few minutes or until the dizziness lessens.

Weight Gain

Chakra: Throat, Solar Plexus, Root

Weight gain may be caused by hormonal issues, eating disorders, or thyroid problems. Therefore, it's important to treat areas associated with weight gain. For unexplained weight gain, suggest your client seek a medical evaluation to ensure they don't have a thyroid disorder.

- Throat hand position supports thyroid, stimulates metabolism, and balances Throat chakra
- Solar Plexus hand position supports self-esteem and balances Solar Plexus chakra
- Groin hand position fights addictions and balances Root chakra

SEQUENCE

1. *Touch:* Throat
2. *Touch:* Solar Plexus
3. *Touch:* Groin

OTHER TECHNIQUES

Recommend your client carry amethyst crystals or wear a piece of amethyst jewelry.

Mental, Emotional, and Spiritual Healing

It is difficult when dealing with a whole human being to separate physical, mental, emotional, and spiritual health. Each affects the others, making up the overall health of an individual. Therefore, when working with a client's health problems, it's also important to work with emotional, mental, and spiritual issues. As with physical problems, these issues can be related to energetic imbalances in the chakras, as well as throughout the subtle (energetic) body.

Optimal health and function requires energetic balance, as well as attention to body, mind, and spirit. Reiki deals with all four of these facets of health. This differs from medical science, which separates physical health from mental, emotional, and spiritual health. As Reiki practitioners, we work with people holistically, seeing them as souls with a body, mind, and spirit that all need to function in balance.

Although mental, emotional, and spiritual issues are separated in medical science from physical health, it's still important to recommend that your clients seek the appropriate physical or mental health care if they are struggling with issues such as severe mood swings (which may be related to a chemical imbalance, as in bipolar disorder), depression, suicidal ideation, and similar issues. As with physical problems, your role is not to diagnose, nor should you contradict recommendations by medical or mental health professionals. Instead, consider your therapy as complementary energetic treatment, offered in conjunction with appropriate physical and mental health care.

In the sections that follow, I've identified common mental, emotional, and spiritual issues, and offer Reiki and other energetic therapies to help balance energies that are frequently associated with them.

Abandonment

Chakra: Root, Sacral

Abandonment feels like betrayal, and the earlier in life someone experiences it, the more likely it is to strongly affect the psyche. Abandonment affects two chakras: abandonment by (or of) family is a Root chakra issue, while abandonment by (or of) partners affects the Sacral chakra. Regardless of whether it's a fear of abandonment, unresolved feelings from abandonment, or a tendency to abandon others in your life, Reiki can help balance energies and bring about healing.

- Heart hand position supports grief arising from abandonment and spurs compassion for people who have a tendency to abandon others
- Solar Plexus hand position supports self-worth and self-esteem issues caused by abandonment
- Navel and Hara hand positions balance Sacral chakra
- Groin hand position balances Root chakra
- Feet hand position provides grounding

SEQUENCE

1. *Touch:* Heart
2. *Touch:* Solar Plexus
3. *Touch:* Navel or Hara
4. *Touch:* Groin
5. *Touch:* Feet

OTHER TECHNIQUES

Place pieces of red-orange carnelian on the treatment table at Hara level on each side of your client.

Abundance, Prosperity

Chakra: Sacral, Root, Solar Plexus

Prosperity issues originate in the Sacral chakra. However, if abundance and prosperity issues are so severe that they affect safety, security, and well-being, they also affect the energy of the Root chakra. When abundance issues affect or arise from lack of self-esteem, they also can cause or be caused by energetic imbalances in the Solar Plexus chakra.

- Solar Plexus hand position balances Solar Plexus chakra and supports self-worth and self-esteem issues caused by lack of abundance
- Navel and Hara hand positions balance Sacral chakra
- Groin hand position improves sense of safety and security and balances Root chakra

SEQUENCE

1. *Touch:* Solar Plexus
2. *Touch:* Navel
3. *Touch:* Hara
4. *Touch:* Groin

OTHER TECHNIQUES

Beliefs about money are often the largest block to prosperity. Have your client affirm daily, "I give thanks that I am abundant in all things," to reverse negative beliefs about abundance.

Abuse

Chakra: Heart, Solar Plexus, Sacral, Root

Abuse—whether as one who was abused or one who abuses—affects the first four chakras. Safety and security issues (Root chakra) are often part of the problem, both in cases of one who is abused and one who abuses. The need to be in control or fear of being controlled (Sacral chakra) and self-worth (Solar Plexus chakra) also play a role in abuse. Finally, the Heart chakra is the place where love, forgiveness, and compassion arise, whether for self or others, all of which are important components in overcoming abuse.

- Throat hand position supports speaking one's truth
- Heart hand position fosters compassion, forgiveness, and unconditional love and balances Heart chakra
- Solar Plexus hand position fosters self-compassion, self-love, and self-worth and balances Solar Plexus chakra
- Adrenals hand position balances adrenal glands
- Navel and Hara hand positions balance Sacral chakra
- Groin hand position balances Root chakra
- Feet hand position encourages self-support

SEQUENCE

1. *Touch:* Throat
2. *Touch:* Heart
3. *Touch:* Adrenals
4. *Touch:* Solar Plexus
5. *Touch:* Navel
6. *Touch:* Hara
7. *Touch:* Groin
8. *Touch:* Feet

OTHER TECHNIQUES

Ruby in fuchsite supports both Root and Heart chakras. Recommend your client wear ruby in fuchsite as a bracelet or ring.

Acceptance, Surrender

Chakra: Solar Plexus, Throat, Root

Acceptance and surrender (or the inability to accept and surrender) are related. Many people struggle with acceptance (Solar Plexus chakra) and the ability to surrender to divine will (Throat chakra). The Root chakra is where one begins to accept oneself as individual from others.

- Throat hand position supports surrender to divine will and balances Throat chakra
- Heart hand position invites compassion
- Solar Plexus hand position fosters self-acceptance and balances Solar Plexus chakra
- Groin hand position supports Root chakra
- Navel hand position improves a sense of self, honesty, and integrity and balances the Sacral chakra

SEQUENCE

1. *Touch:* Throat
2. *Touch:* Heart
3. *Touch:* Solar Plexus
4. *Touch:* Navel
5. *Touch:* Groin

OTHER TECHNIQUES

Place a piece of blue calcite on your client's Throat chakra.

Addiction

Chakra: Root

Although addiction problems originate energetically in the Root chakra, other areas and chakras are also affected.

- Throat hand position supports surrendering personal will to divine will (or a higher power)
- Heart hand position invites love, compassion, and forgiveness
- Adrenals hand position fights adrenal exhaustion and fatigue
- Solar Plexus hand position fosters personal responsibility and stimulates willpower
- Groin hand position balances Root chakra
- Feet hand position helps grounding, which can be an issue in addiction

SEQUENCE

1. *Touch:* Throat
2. *Touch:* Heart
3. *Touch:* Adrenals
4. *Touch:* Solar Plexus
5. *Touch:* Groin
6. *Touch:* Feet

OTHER TECHNIQUES

Amethyst is considered the sober stone, and it is often used in energetic treatment of all types of addiction. Recommend your client wear amethyst jewelry or carry a piece of amethyst.

Anger, Rage, Resentment, Bitterness

Chakra: Heart

When anger is chronic or the go-to emotion, or when one can't control it, then it's a problem. Rage, anger, and resentment are all degrees on the same scale. Rage is the most severe form of anger, while resentment arises when anger simmers unresolved for a long period. Bitterness is the end result of simmering anger or resentment. Unbalanced energy of the Heart chakra contributes to anger energy.

- Throat hand position supports speaking one's truth and expressing anger appropriately
- Heart hand position balances Heart chakra
- Adrenals hand position (palms on rib cage under breasts, with fingertips pointed toward sternum) supports adrenals
- Solar Plexus hand position fosters self-worth and self-esteem

SEQUENCE

1. *Touch:* Throat
2. *Touch:* Heart
3. *Touch:* Adrenals
4. *Touch:* Solar Plexus

OTHER TECHNIQUES

Your client can perform the following meditation when they feel themselves experiencing any of these emotions for five minutes or as long as it takes to feel peace. The client sits with their feet flat on the floor, breathing in deeply through the nose and out through the mouth. The client visualizes peace coming in through their nose, filling their lungs, and traveling throughout their body. They visualize anger gathering in the center of the chest and draining out through the feet into the Earth. As they do this, the client repeats the mantra, "I breathe in peace. I release all anger."

Anxiety, Fear, Worry, Stress, Panic

Chakra: Root

It's natural to feel anxious or afraid occasionally. Humans are programmed with a fight-or-flight instinct as a response to fear to protect us from predators. Unfortunately, many people experience chronic stress, fear, worry, or anxiety. These are all degrees on the same scale. When fear becomes chronic, it manifests as stress, worry, and anxiety. These issues are generally related to safety and security (Root chakra). Chronic anxiety also affects the adrenal glands and can lead to adrenal fatigue.

- Throat hand position supports thyroid hormones (imbalances of these hormones may contribute to anxiety)
- Adrenals hand position supports adrenal glands
- Hara and Groin hand positions balance Root chakra

SEQUENCE

1. *Touch:* Throat
2. *Touch:* Adrenals
3. *Touch:* Hara
4. *Touch:* Groin

OTHER TECHNIQUES

Recommend that when your client notices feelings of fear, they close their eyes and focus on breathing in through the nose, repeating, "I breathe in peace." Then exhale through the mouth, repeating, "I exhale fear." They can do this for a few moments or until they start to feel calmer.

Centering

Chakra: Solar Plexus, Heart, Throat

Being centered can help one remain calm in stressful situations and grounded in times of great emotion or difficulty, as well as maintain focus and clarity. The Heart chakra is the center chakra of the seven main chakras and bridges body and spirit. Along with the heart, bringing energy to and balancing the Throat and Solar Plexus chakras can help with centering.

- Throat hand position draws energy downward from upper chakras toward Heart chakra
- Solar Plexus hand position draws energy upward from lower chakras toward Heart chakra
- Heart hand position centers energy

SEQUENCE

1. *Touch:* Throat chakra and Solar Plexus chakra simultaneously, one hand on each
2. *Touch:* Heart

OTHER TECHNIQUES

Your client can use the following meditation on their own when they feel out of balance for a few minutes or until they feel centered: The client places their hands over the Hara and breathes deeply, feeling the breath move under their hands and visualizing a warm, pink ball of light growing in the Hara under their hands.

Communication, Self-Expression

Chakra: Throat

Clear communication is essential not only to human relationships, but also to how we express ourselves creatively and our ability to speak and understand our own personal truths. The Throat chakra is the center of communication, while the Third Eye chakra facilitates communication with our higher selves and receptiveness to divine guidance. Meanwhile, the Sacral chakra sparks creative ideas that can help us communicate.

- Throat hand position facilitates clear communication and balances the Throat chakra
- Eyes hand position allows divine guidance and balances the Third Eye chakra
- Ears hand position facilitates listening and balances the Third Eye chakra
- Hara hand position sparks creativity in communication and balances the Sacral chakra

SEQUENCE

1. *Touch:* Eyes
2. *Touch:* Ears
3. *Touch:* Hara
4. *Touch:* Throat

OTHER TECHNIQUES

Recommend your client affirm daily, "I clearly hear what others are saying, and I communicate clearly and concisely."

Compassion, Kindness

Chakra: Heart

To live with kindness and compassion, one must approach the world with gentleness, release judgment of self and others, and wish to be a force of light and goodness in daily life. All of us occasionally fail to act with kindness and compassion, but a habitual lack of these qualities may be related to energetic imbalances in the Heart chakra.

- Eyes hand position connects with a higher power to inspire compassion
- Ears hand position supports listening and hearing with compassion
- Throat hand position facilitates communication with compassion
- Heart hand position balances Heart chakra and fosters unconditional love
- Solar Plexus hand position fosters compassion for self

SEQUENCE

1. *Touch:* Eyes
2. *Touch:* Ears
3. *Touch:* Throat
4. *Touch:* Heart
5. *Touch:* Solar Plexus

OTHER TECHNIQUES

Rose quartz, kunzite, and morganite are stones of compassion that support the Heart chakra. Your client can use the following meditation on their own for five minutes or for as long as they feel comfortable doing so: Holding one of these stones to the Heart chakra, the client visualizes the energy of love emanating from the stone as a pink light. They visualize light entering the body through the Heart chakra, where it moves into the heart. The client visualizes the heart pumping pink light throughout the body.

Concentration, Clarity, Focus (and Confusion)

Chakra: Third Eye

Concentration, focus, and clarity are all matters of the mind and spirit. Whether one wishes to receive clarity from the higher self or the divine or to achieve concentration and clarity in thinking, focusing on the Third Eye chakra is helpful in balancing energies. This treatment can also help alleviate confusion.

- Eyes, Ears, and Back of Head hand positions balance Third Eye chakra

SEQUENCE

1. *Touch:* Eyes
2. *Tap:* Two-finger tap on the third eye in a counterclockwise circle
3. *Touch:* Ears
4. *Touch:* Back of Head

OTHER TECHNIQUES

Calcite stones are known as "student stones" because they enhance focus and concentration. Place pieces of blue calcite on the treatment table on each side of your client's head.

Confidence

Chakra: Solar Plexus, Root

Confidence arises from a strong sense of self, and balancing the energy of the Solar Plexus chakra can assist with this. However, it is difficult to have confidence if safety and security (Root chakra) issues are not addressed first.

- Hara and Groin hand positions balance Root chakra
- Knees and Feet hand positions support independent action (standing on one's own two feet)
- Solar Plexus hand position supports self-confidence and self-worth and balances Solar Plexus chakra

SEQUENCE

1. *Touch:* Hara
2. *Touch:* Groin
3. *Stroke:* Stroke palms from tops of thighs down front of legs to tops of knees
4. *Touch:* Knees
5. *Stroke:* Stroke palms down along the shins, from base of the knees to ankles
6. *Touch:* Feet
7. *Touch:* Solar Plexus

OTHER TECHNIQUES

Yellow tiger's eye is a stone of strength, will, and empowerment. Recommend your client carry a piece of yellow tiger's eye in their front pocket or wear it in a bracelet or necklace.

Courage

Chakra: Solar Plexus, Root

Courage is acting despite being afraid to do so. This trait isn't limited to acts of valor, but also to the small daily acts that require bravery in the face of anxieties, fears, and worries. Unbalanced Solar Plexus chakra energies may contribute to a lack of courage, and rebalancing these energies can help one be more courageous— not just for the big things, but also for the small acts of bravery in daily life. Increasing a sense of safety and security (Root chakra) can also inspire more courage.

- Hara and Groin hand positions balance Root chakra
- Knees, Ankles, and Feet hand positions support independent action (standing on one's own two feet)
- Solar Plexus hand position supports courage

SEQUENCE

1. *Touch:* Hara
2. *Touch:* Groin
3. *Touch:* Knees
4. *Touch:* Ankles
5. *Touch:* Feet
6. *Touch:* Solar Plexus

OTHER TECHNIQUES

Place a yellow tiger's eye pyramid under the treatment table with the point in line with the Solar Plexus chakra.

Creativity, Inspiration

Chakra: Third Eye, Throat, Sacral

Many people (including me) believe all inspiration and creativity come from higher realms. Therefore, stimulating the Third Eye chakra can spark creativity. From a chakra perspective, creative energy arises from the Sacral chakra, while the power to express creative ideas comes from balanced energies of the Throat chakra.

- Eyes hand position stimulates Third Eye chakra
- Ears hand position allows you to hear and receive creative inspiration
- Throat hand position supports creative expression and balances the Throat chakra
- Solar Plexus hand position provides self-confidence to move forward with creative ideas
- Navel and Hara hand positions support creativity and balance the Sacral chakra

SEQUENCE

1. *Touch:* Eyes
2. *Tap:* Two-finger tap along brows
3. *Touch:* Ears
4. *Touch:* Navel
5. *Touch:* Hara
6. *Touch:* Solar Plexus
7. *Touch:* Throat

OTHER TECHNIQUES

Place a piece of rainbow fluorite under the treatment table.

Denial, Letting Go

Chakra: Sacral

Denial and the inability to let go arise from the desire to control self, others, emotions, situations, and circumstances (Sacral chakra). It is difficult for many people to learn to let go, because doing so is jumping into the unknown and trusting that if you fall, someone will catch you (or you'll catch yourself).

- Solar Plexus hand position strengthens personal will
- Navel and Hara hand positions balance Sacral chakra
- Groin hand position promotes safety and security

SEQUENCE

1. *Touch:* Solar Plexus
2. *Touch:* Groin
3. *Touch:* Navel
4. *Touch:* Hara

OTHER TECHNIQUES

You can teach your client the following meditation to use on their own when they are having difficulty letting go. They can do this for five minutes or as long as they feel necessary. The client sits in a chair with their feet flat on the floor, breathing deeply through the nose and visualizing inhaling peace and trust. Then, they breathe out forcefully through the mouth to quickly expel all the air, as they say in their mind, "Release" or "Let go."

Depression

Chakra: Root, Third Eye, Sacral

Depression is sadness that lingers. It can be temporary, based on circumstances, or it can be a chemical reaction related to neurotransmitters in the brain. The energy of depression comes from imbalances in the Root chakra, but focusing on the nervous system (Third Eye chakra), where neurotransmitters are produced, stored, and released, can also help. The Sacral chakra strengthens personal will and can help balance hormonal issues that may be associated with depression.

- Groin hand position balances Root chakra
- Hara hand position balances Sacral chakra
- Heart hand position facilitates love
- Eyes, Ears, and Back of Head hand positions support nervous system and balance Third Eye chakra

SEQUENCE

1. *Touch:* Groin
2. *Touch:* Hara
3. *Touch:* Heart
4. *Touch:* Eyes
5. *Touch:* Ears
6. *Touch:* Back of Head

OTHER TECHNIQUES

Recommend your client wear a yellow Baltic amber bracelet or ring during episodes of depression.

Dreams

Chakra: Third Eye, Crown

Dreaming offers guidance from the higher self and the divine. Supporting the upper chakras can help alleviate nightmares and support dreams that provide important messages.

- Eyes, Ears, and Back of Head hand positions balance Crown and Third Eye chakras

SEQUENCE

1. *Touch:* Eyes
2. *Tap:* Two-finger tap directly on Third Eye chakra in a counterclockwise motion
3. *Touch:* Ears
4. *Touch:* Back of Head

OTHER TECHNIQUES

Recommend your client sleep with amethyst on a bedside table.

Empathy

Chakra: Heart, Third Eye, Crown

Empathy, or the ability to put oneself emotionally in someone else's shoes, originates in the Heart chakra as a function of unconditional love. Some people are also naturally empathic, which is a form of psychic energy where someone experiences the emotions (and sometimes physical symptoms) of others as their own. Whether the problem is too little empathy or too much, the ways to balance the energy are the same. The Crown and Third Eye chakras can bring higher guidance, which can help with empathy.

- Heart hand position balances empathy and Heart chakra and stimulates unconditional love
- Eyes hand position balances Third Eye and Crown chakras
- Groin and Feet hand positions facilitate grounding, which can help over-empathizers

SEQUENCE

1. *Touch:* Eyes
2. *Touch:* Heart (if overly empathic, go to step three; if lacking empathy, remain on the heart for three more minutes and then go to step four)
3. *Touch:* Groin
4. *Touch:* Feet

OTHER TECHNIQUES

Opaque crystals absorb excess energy, while translucent crystals amplify it. For over-empathizers, suggest they carry with them an opaque green stone, such as green aventurine or amazonite, which can help absorb excess heart energy. For under-empathizers, suggest they carry with them a transparent green stone, such as peridot or green fluorite, to help amplify heart energy.

Empowerment

Chakra: Root, Solar Plexus, Throat

Empowerment energy starts in the Root chakra, where one develops the ability to stand on one's own two feet and grow in safety and security. In the Solar Plexus chakra, empowerment energy continues to develop with self-identity and self-confidence. In the Throat chakra, empowerment continues with the ability to express oneself and speak the truth.

- Feet and Knees hand positions support independent action (standing on one's own two feet) while remaining grounded
- Groin hand position balances Root chakra
- Solar Plexus hand position develops a sense of self-empowerment, will, and self-worth and balances the Solar Plexus chakra
- Throat hand position facilitates speaking and communicating truth from a strong and empowered place and balances the Throat chakra

SEQUENCE

1. *Touch:* Feet
2. *Touch:* Knees
3. *Touch:* Groin
4. *Touch:* Solar Plexus
5. *Touch:* Throat

OTHER TECHNIQUES

Use a chakra-balancing program or smartphone app; these tools play tones that start in the Root chakra and run up to the Crown chakra.

Faith, Optimism, Hope

Chakra: Solar Plexus, Third Eye, Crown

Most people associate faith with belief in a higher power, but it can also be faith in yourself, in other people, in the greater good, or in the kindness of strangers. Faith is the cousin of optimism and hope, and all three can be strengthened by balancing the energy of the Solar Plexus, Third Eye, and Crown chakras.

- Solar Plexus hand position supports self-esteem and balances the Solar Plexus chakra
- Heart hand position supports optimism and unconditional love
- Throat hand position supports surrender of personal will to divine will
- Eyes and Ears hand positions balance Crown and Third Eye chakras

SEQUENCE

1. *Touch:* Solar Plexus
2. *Touch:* Heart
3. *Touch:* Throat
4. *Touch:* Eyes
5. *Touch:* Ears

OTHER TECHNIQUES

With you or on their own, encourage your client to chant the Bija mantra for the Third Eye chakra, which is OM (pronounced *ohm*). (Bija are special mantras that have the power to create transformative energy.)

Forgiveness

Chakra: Heart

Many people misunderstand forgiveness, believing "to forgive" means absolving another for their actions. In fact, forgiveness is always about the person doing the forgiving and never about the person being forgiven. The act of forgiveness is stating the other person's actions no longer have any power over you.

- Heart hand position balances the Heart chakra.

SEQUENCE

1. *Touch:* Heart

OTHER TECHNIQUES

Visualization is a powerful path to forgiveness. Your client can do the following self-guided meditation for five minutes or longer as needed. The client closes their eyes and visualizes themselves and the person they wish to forgive, seeing the ties between them as glowing strands of energy. Once the client sees those clearly, they use imaginary scissors to cut those energetic strands, saying silently or aloud, "I release you."

Gratitude

Chakra: Heart

Living with gratitude has many benefits, including increased happiness, joy, compassion, and kindness. It is primarily a function of the Heart chakra.

- Heart hand position supports love and gratitude and balances the Heart chakra
- Hara hand position pulls energy through the lower chakras
- Eyes and Ears hand positions pull energy through the upper chakras

SEQUENCE

1. *Touch:* Heart
2. *Touch:* Hara and Third Eye chakra simultaneously, one hand on each

OTHER TECHNIQUES

Suggest your client start or end each day by listing things for which they are grateful.

Grief

Chakra: Heart

Grief lingers in the Heart chakra, and balancing Heart chakra energy can help resolve it over time.

- Heart hand position balances Heart chakra
- Adrenals hand position supports adrenal fatigue associated with grief
- Throat hand position supports expression of grief

SEQUENCE

1. *Touch:* Throat
2. *Touch:* Heart
3. *Touch:* Adrenals
4. *Touch:* Heart

OTHER TECHNIQUES

Place pieces of Apache tears on the treatment table on each side of your client's Heart chakra.

Grounding

Chakra: Root

Grounding helps one stay focused on the here and now. It can help whenever one is overcome with powerful emotions, as well.

- Groin hand position balances Root chakra
- Knees, Ankles, and Feet hand positions are grounding

SEQUENCE

1. *Touch:* Groin
2. *Touch:* Knees
3. *Touch:* Ankles
4. *Touch:* Feet

OTHER TECHNIQUES

Suggest that whenever your client feels ungrounded, they sit in a chair and place their feet flat on the floor, visualizing roots growing into the Earth from the bottoms of their feet for a few minutes.

Guilt, Shame

Chakra: Solar Plexus

Guilt and shame are degrees of feeling along the same scale. Guilt is a passing feeling, while shame is deeply entrenched. Unbalanced Solar Plexus chakra energy contributes to guilt and shame.

- Solar Plexus and Middle Back (with client lying facedown) hand positions balance Solar Plexus chakra
- Heart hand position fosters self-forgiveness

SEQUENCE

1. *Touch:* Solar Plexus
2. *Touch:* Heart
3. *Touch:* Middle Back (with client lying facedown)

OTHER TECHNIQUES

Whenever your client experiences guilt and shame, they can use the following technique for five minutes or as long as they would like. The client visualizes shame or guilt in the Solar Plexus chakra and imagines pulling the energy into their heart to heal it with love.

Indecisiveness

Chakra: Sacral, Solar Plexus, Third Eye

To be decisive, one must know what they want and have a sense of self (Sacral chakra) as well as the self-confidence to make a decision (Solar Plexus chakra). Higher guidance (Third Eye chakra) can also help in decision-making.

- Hara and Navel hand positions balance Sacral chakra
- Solar Plexus hand position balances Solar Plexus chakra
- Eyes hand position supports higher guidance and balances Third Eye chakra

SEQUENCE

1. *Touch:* Hara
2. *Touch:* Navel
3. *Touch:* Solar Plexus
4. *Touch:* Eyes

OTHER TECHNIQUES

Suggest that a client who is struggling with a difficult decision request before going to sleep at night, "Tell me what I need to know." Then, advise them to pay attention to what arises in their dreams, as dreams often provide symbolic or literal information to help one understand their path.

Insecurity

Chakra: Root, Solar Plexus

Basic safety and security (Root chakra) are necessary before one can become personally secure and develop a sense of self-esteem and self-worth (Solar Plexus chakra).

- Feet, Ankles, and Knees hand positions support independent action (standing on one's own two feet)
- Groin hand position balances Root chakra
- Solar Plexus hand position balances Solar Plexus chakra

SEQUENCE

1. *Touch:* Feet
2. *Touch:* Ankles
3. *Touch:* Knees
4. *Touch:* Groin
5. *Touch:* Solar Plexus

OTHER TECHNIQUES

Place a piece of red tiger's eye between your client's legs on the treatment table and yellow tiger's eye under the table at the level of the Solar Plexus chakra.

Insomnia, Sleeplessness

Chakra: Third Eye, Crown

Difficulty sleeping comes from Crown and Third Eye chakra imbalances and may also be related to thyroid (Throat chakra) and adrenal (Solar Plexus chakra) imbalances.

- Solar Plexus hand position balances adrenal glands and Solar Plexus chakra
- Adrenals hand position supports adrenal glands
- Throat hand position supports thyroid and balances Throat chakra
- Eyes, Ears, and Back of Head hand positions support Crown and Third Eye chakras

SEQUENCE

1. *Touch:* Solar Plexus
2. *Touch:* Adrenals
3. *Touch:* Throat
4. *Touch:* Eyes
5. *Touch:* Ears
6. *Touch:* Back of Head

OTHER TECHNIQUES

- Diffuse lavender essential oil during the session.
- Recommend your client sleep with a piece of amethyst on their bedside table.

Intuition

Chakra: Third Eye, Crown

Intuition comes from the higher self and the divine, which enter the mind through the Third Eye and Crown chakras.

- Eyes, Ears, and Back of Head hand positions support Crown and Third Eye chakras

SEQUENCE

1. *Touch:* Eyes
2. *Tap:* Two-finger tap around Third Eye chakra in counterclockwise motion
3. *Touch:* Ears
4. *Touch:* Back of Head

OTHER TECHNIQUES

Place pieces of clear quartz on the treatment table on each side of your client's head.

Irritability

Chakra: Solar Plexus, Sacral, Root

Irritability tends to originate in the Solar Plexus, Sacral, and Root chakras, where issues of security, safety, self-identity, and self-worth come into play. Hormonally, the thyroid (Throat chakra) and adrenal glands may also play a role.

- Heart hand position strengthens compassion, and centers and balances the Heart Chakra
- Groin hand position balances Root chakra
- Hara and Navel hand positions balance Sacral chakra
- Adrenals hand position supports adrenal glands
- Solar Plexus hand position balances Solar Plexus chakra
- Throat hand position supports thyroid and balances Throat chakra

SEQUENCE

1. *Touch:* Groin
2. *Touch:* Hara
3. *Touch:* Navel
4. *Touch:* Adrenals
5. *Touch:* Solar Plexus
6. *Touch:* Throat
7. *Touch:* Heart

OTHER TECHNIQUES

Blue lace agate supplies calming energy. Place a piece of blue lace agate near your client's throat on the treatment table.

Joy, Happiness

Chakra: Sacral, Heart

Joy originates in Sacral chakra energy, but moving into a place of love (Heart chakra) can also support happiness.

- Hara and Navel hand positions balance Sacral chakra
- Heart hand position supports unconditional love and balances Heart chakra

SEQUENCE

1. *Touch:* Hara
2. *Touch:* Navel
3. *Touch:* Heart

OTHER TECHNIQUES

During treatment, have your client visualize breathing in joy through the nose as a bright orange light for as long as feels comfortable.

Laziness

Chakra: Root

When energy remains blocked in the Root chakra, laziness can result. Therefore, supporting this chakra is essential in curing laziness.

- Hara, Groin, and Tops of Legs (with client lying facedown) hand positions balance Root chakra

SEQUENCE

1. *Touch:* Hara
2. *Touch:* Groin
3. *Touch:* Tops of Legs (with client lying facedown)

OTHER TECHNIQUES

Place a piece of red garnet on the treatment table between your client's legs.

Loneliness

Chakra: Heart, Solar Plexus, Sacral

People who are lonely often have difficulty opening their hearts (Heart chakra) to others. They may also suffer from lack of self-esteem and self-identity (Solar Plexus and Sacral chakras).

- Hara and Navel hand positions balance Sacral chakra
- Solar Plexus hand position balances Solar Plexus chakra
- Heart hand position supports unconditional love and balances Heart chakra

SEQUENCE

1. *Touch:* Hara
2. *Touch:* Navel
3. *Touch:* Solar Plexus
4. *Touch:* Heart

OTHER TECHNIQUES

Place a piece of morganite over your client's Heart chakra.

Love

Chakra: Heart

Whether it's romantic, familial, friendly, or unconditional love, all love originates in the Heart chakra. Balancing the energies here will foster love.

- Heart and Middle Back (with client lying facedown) hand positions foster and strengthen love and balance Heart chakra
- Solar Plexus hand position fosters self-love and balances Heart chakra

SEQUENCE

1. *Touch:* Solar Plexus
2. *Touch:* Heart
3. *Touch:* Middle Back (with client lying facedown)

OTHER TECHNIQUES

Place pieces of rose quartz on the treatment table on each side of your client's Heart chakra.

Luck, Optimism

Chakra: Solar Plexus, Throat, Third Eye

In metaphysical circles, we tend to believe you make your own luck through positive thinking (Third Eye chakra), visualization, positive communication (Throat chakra), and remaining focused on what you desire. Good luck and optimism energy originate in the Solar Plexus chakra and travel upward.

- Solar Plexus hand position balances Solar Plexus chakra
- Throat hand position supports optimistic communication and balances Heart chakra
- Back of Head, Ears, and Eyes hand positions foster positive thinking and balance the Third Eye chakra

SEQUENCE

1. *Touch:* Solar Plexus
2. *Touch:* Throat
3. *Touch:* Back of Head
4. *Touch:* Ears
5. *Touch:* Eyes

OTHER TECHNIQUES

Place a piece of green aventurine under the treatment table.

Memory

Chakra: Third Eye

Memory is a function of brainpower, which originates in the Third Eye chakra.

- Eyes, Ears, and Back of Head hand positions support Third Eye chakra

SEQUENCE

1. *Touch:* Eyes
2. *Tap:* Two-finger tap of Third Eye chakra in counterclockwise circle
3. *Touch:* Ears
4. *Touch:* Back of Head

OTHER TECHNIQUES

Diffuse rosemary essential oil during the session.

Mood Swings

Chakra: Heart, Throat, Solar Plexus, Sacral

Mood swings may be the result of hormonal issues from sex hormones (Sacral chakra), thyroid (Throat chakra), or adrenals (Solar Plexus chakra). They may also be related to a lack of self-esteem or to anger or bitterness (Heart chakra).

- Hara and Navel hand positions support Sacral chakra
- Adrenals hand position supports adrenal glands
- Solar Plexus hand position supports self-esteem and Solar Plexus chakra
- Heart hand position dispels anger and supports Heart chakra
- Throat hand position supports thyroid and Throat chakra

SEQUENCE

1. *Touch:* Hara
2. *Touch:* Navel
3. *Touch:* Adrenals
4. *Touch:* Solar Plexus
5. *Touch:* Throat
6. *Touch:* Heart

OTHER TECHNIQUES

Recommend your client wear rose quartz jewelry or carry a piece of rose quartz for a calming effect.

Motivation

Chakra: Solar Plexus

Motivation comes from self-worth, which originates in the Solar Plexus chakra. However, you may also want to pump up the desire to "get up and go" by working from the feet up to the groin, moving the energy upward to the Solar Plexus chakra.

- Feet, Ankles, Knees, Groin, Hara, and Navel hand positions move energy upward from the Earth to help client "get up"

- Solar Plexus hand position balances Solar Plexus chakra

SEQUENCE

1. *Touch:* Feet
2. *Touch:* Ankles
3. *Stroke:* Stroke palms up along shins from ankles to knees
4. *Touch:* Knees
5. *Stroke:* Stroke palms up along fronts of thighs from tops of knees to tops of thighs
6. *Touch:* Groin
7. *Touch:* Hara
8. *Touch:* Navel
9. *Touch:* Solar Plexus

OTHER TECHNIQUES

Place a piece of carnelian on the treatment table on each side of your client's Sacral chakra.

Negativity, Judgment

Chakra: Throat

Negativity and judgment originate in the Throat chakra, where one gives expression to thoughts, beliefs, and judgments. Moving this energy downward into the heart can help replace negativity and judgment with love.

- Throat hand position balances Throat chakra
- Heart hand position brings love into the situation

SEQUENCE

1. *Touch:* Throat
2. *Touch:* Heart

OTHER TECHNIQUES

Diffuse lemon essential oil during the session.

Obsession, Compulsion

Chakra: Root, Sacral

Obsession and compulsion energies originate in Root chakra imbalances. However, these issues are also about control, which is a Sacral chakra issue.

- Groin and Tops of Legs (with client lying facedown) hand positions balance Root chakra
- Hara, Navel, and Lower Back (with client lying facedown) hand positions balance Sacral chakra

SEQUENCE

1. *Touch:* Groin
2. *Touch:* Hara
3. *Touch:* Navel
4. *Touch:* Tops of Legs (with client lying facedown)
5. *Touch:* Lower Back (with client lying facedown)

OTHER TECHNIQUES

Second-degree practitioners can draw SHK over the Root, Sacral, and Solar Plexus chakras to release energy associated with obsessions and compulsions.

Overindulgence

Chakra: Solar Plexus

Everyone overindulges from time to time, but if it becomes chronic, it can be a problem. Overindulgence arises from a lack of self-control, which is a Solar Plexus chakra issue.

- Solar Plexus hand position balances the Solar Plexus chakra
- Navel, Hara, Groin, Knees, Ankles, and Feet hand positions draw the energy of overindulgence downward and discharge it into the Earth

SEQUENCE

1. *Touch:* Navel
2. *Touch:* Hara
3. *Touch:* Groin
4. *Stroke:* Stroke palms downward from tops of thighs to tops of knees
5. *Touch:* Knees
6. *Stroke:* Stroke palms downward along shins from knees to ankles
7. *Touch:* Ankles
8. *Touch:* Feet
9. *Touch:* Solar Plexus

OTHER TECHNIQUES

Place a piece of tiger's eye on your client's Solar Plexus chakra.

Passion

Chakra: Root, Sacral

Passion ignites when energy travels up from the Root chakra and into the Sacral chakra.

- Groin and Tops of Legs (with client lying facedown) hand positions stimulate Root chakra energy
- Navel, Hara, and Lower Back (with client lying facedown) hand positions stimulate Sacral chakra energy

SEQUENCE

1. *Touch:* Groin
2. *Touch:* Navel
3. *Touch:* Hara
4. *Touch:* Tops of Legs (with client lying facedown)
5. *Touch:* Lower Back (with client lying facedown)

OTHER TECHNIQUES

Place a piece of garnet on the treatment table between your client's legs.

Peace

Chakra: Heart

The feeling of peace originates in the Heart chakra and emanates outward from there.

- Heart hand position balances Heart chakra
- Throat, Eyes, Ears, and Back of Head hand positions draw peace upward
- Solar Plexus, Hara, and Groin hand positions draw peace downward

SEQUENCE

1. *Touch:* Heart
2. *Touch:* Solar Plexus
3. *Touch:* Hara
4. *Touch:* Groin
5. *Touch:* Heart
6. *Touch:* Throat
7. *Touch:* Back of Head
8. *Touch:* Ears
9. *Touch:* Eyes
10. *Touch:* Heart

OTHER TECHNIQUES

Place a piece of kunzite or rose quartz on your client's Heart chakra.

Phobias

Chakra: Root

Phobias are a form of anxiety or fear, which originate in the Root chakra.

- Groin and Tops of Legs (with client lying facedown) hand positions balance Root chakra
- Knees, Ankles, and Feet draw fear energy downward to be neutralized by the Earth

SEQUENCE

1. *Touch:* Groin
2. *Stroke:* Stroke palms downward along fronts of thighs from tops of thighs to knees
3. *Touch:* Knees
4. *Stroke:* Stroke palms downward along shins from bottoms of knees to ankles
5. *Touch:* Ankles
6. *Touch:* Feet
7. *Stroke:* With client lying facedown, stroke palms upward along backs of legs from ankles up to bottom of buttocks
8. *Touch:* Tops of Legs (with client lying facedown)

OTHER TECHNIQUES

Second-degree practitioners can draw CKR + SHK + CKR along the client's lower body to release phobia energy that is stuck.

Repression

Chakra: Throat

Repression is lack of expression, which originates in the Throat chakra. Imbalances there may keep one from speaking their truth. A secondary focus on the Solar Plexus chakra for self-worth and the Heart chakra for communicating with love also helps.

- Throat hand position balances Throat chakra
- Heart hand position brings love and balances Heart chakra
- Solar Plexus hand position supports self-worth and balances Solar Plexus chakra

SEQUENCE

1. *Touch:* Throat
2. *Touch:* Solar Plexus
3. *Touch:* Heart

OTHER TECHNIQUES

Place a piece of sodalite on the treatment table on each side of your client's Throat chakra.

Self-Control, Willpower

Chakra: Solar Plexus

Willpower and self-control come from strength of will, which originates with balanced energy in the Solar Plexus chakra.

- Solar Plexus and Middle Back (with client lying facedown) hand positions balance Solar Plexus chakra

SEQUENCE

1. *Touch:* Solar Plexus
2. *Touch:* Middle Back (with client lying facedown)

OTHER TECHNIQUES

Place a piece of citrine on the treatment table on each side of your client's solar plexus.

Self-Esteem, Self-Worth

Chakra: Solar Plexus

The energy to support self-esteem and self-worth is in the Solar Plexus chakra. But before one can find these, they must feel safe and secure (Root chakra) and have a sense of self (Sacral chakra).

- Groin hand position supports safety and security and balances Root chakra
- Hara and Navel hand positions support self-identity and balance Sacral chakra
- Solar Plexus hand position balances Solar Plexus chakra

SEQUENCE

1. *Touch:* Groin
2. *Touch:* Hara
3. *Touch:* Navel
4. *Touch:* Solar Plexus

OTHER TECHNIQUES

Whenever your client feels insecure, or as a daily affirmation, suggest they repeat the affirmation, "I am safe, I know who I am, and I love myself unconditionally."

Self-Harm, Self-Sabotage

Chakra: Root

If someone self-harms or habitually self-sabotages, chances are they have blocked or imbalanced Root chakra energy.

- Feet, Ankles, and Knees hand positions draw energy upward from the Earth
- Groin hand position balances Root chakra

SEQUENCE

1. *Touch:* Feet
2. *Touch:* Ankles
3. *Touch:* Knees
4. *Touch:* Groin

OTHER TECHNIQUES

Place a piece of smoky quartz on the treatment table between your client's legs.

Shyness, Social Anxiety

Chakra: Sacral

If your client is extremely shy or experiences social anxiety, it likely results from an imbalance in Sacral chakra energy. Providing support through the Throat chakra for self-expression, Solar Plexus chakra for self-esteem, and Heart chakra for love can also help.

- Hara and Navel hand positions balance Sacral chakra
- Solar Plexus hand position strengthens self-esteem and balances Solar Plexus chakra
- Heart hand position strengthens love and balances Heart chakra
- Throat hand position encourages self-expression and communication and balances Throat chakra

SEQUENCE

1. *Touch:* Hara
2. *Touch:* Navel
3. *Touch:* Solar Plexus
4. *Touch:* Throat
5. *Touch:* Heart
6. *Touch:* Hara

OTHER TECHNIQUES

Place a piece of carnelian under the treatment table at the Hara level.

Trust

Chakra: Root

Trust develops in the Root chakra from feelings of safety and security. If you do not feel safe or secure, you will be unable to trust. Working with Earth energy from the ground up through this chakra can help.

- Feet, Ankles, and Knees hand positions draw energy up from the Earth
- Groin and Tops of Legs (with client lying facedown) hand positions balance Root chakra

SEQUENCE

1. *Touch:* Feet
2. *Touch:* Ankles
3. *Touch:* Knees
4. *Stroke:* Stroke palms up fronts of legs from ankles to groin
5. *Touch:* Groin
6. *Touch:* Tops of Legs (with client lying facedown)

OTHER TECHNIQUES

During treatment, have your client silently repeat the affirmation, "I am safe. I trust in the universe," for as long as they would like. They can also repeat this affirmation whenever they begin to feel unsafe.

Resources

Caroline Myss Chakra Information

Myss.com

Carline Myss has an excellent chakra flash animation (www.myss .com/free-resources/chakras-your-energetic-being) that tells you everything you need to know about the energy of each chakra and associated spiritual, mental, physical, and emotional issues.

International Association of Reiki Professionals (IARP)

IARP.org

An organization for Reiki professionals with member benefits, including articles, training, and a journal.

International Center for Reiki Training

Reiki.org

Website with articles and information about Reiki, its history, and its practices.

Reiki Rays

ReikiRays.com

Excellent website with free Reiki books, articles, and information about hand positions and more.

SHARe Reiki Community Facebook Group

Facebook.com/groups/889280421213997

An informal group for support, advice, fellowship, and ongoing information about Reiki.

BOOKS

***Anatomy of the Spirit* by Caroline Myss (Harmony, 1996)**
I believe this is the single-best guide you can buy about the human energy anatomy and health issues associated with the chakras. It's well written, comprehensive, and well organized.

***Crystals for Beginners* by Karen Frazier (Althea Press, 2017)**
This is a good beginner's guide to crystal energy, which you can use in your Reiki practice as supplemental therapy.

***Essential Reiki* by Diane Stein (Crossing Press, 1995)**
A comprehensive Reiki manual that provides all the information you'll need after being attuned. Many Reiki master-teachers use this as their Reiki manual for students of all three degrees.

***The Reiki Manual* by Penelope Quest and Kathy Roberts (TarcherPerigee, 2011)**
A comprehensive and informative Reiki manual that many Reiki masters offer to their students in all three degrees of Reiki.

***The Subtle Body* by Cyndi Dale (Sounds True, 2009)**
This book offers an encyclopedia of human energy anatomy and is an excellent learning and reference tool. I refer to it regularly.

APPS

Healing Crystals Database
A reasonably comprehensive crystals guide, with crystal information at your fingertips.

Reiki Energy by Vincent Barousse
An excellent app that offers quick treatment for various conditions and a Reiki timer.

Reiki Healing Music Therapy Holistic Massage Music by Rehegoo
An app featuring an assortment of Reiki music with three- and five-minute timers.

References

American Autoimmune Related Diseases Association. "Autoimmune Disease List." Accessed March 5, 2018. https://www.aarda.org/diseaselist/.

Doran, Bernadette. "The Science Behind Reiki." *The Reiki Times,* Summer 2009. www.equilibrium-e3.com/images/PDF/Science%20Behind%20Reiki.pdf.

Ehrlich, George E. "Low Back Pain." *Bulletin of the World Health Organization* 9, no. 81 (2003): 671–676. https://doi.org/10.1001/jama.1982.03330070068042.

Myss, Caroline M. *Anatomy of the Spirit: The Seven Stages of Power and Healing.* New York: Harmony, 1996.

Ramirez, Jonatan Peña, et al. "The Sympathy of Two Pendulum Clocks: Beyond Huygens' Observations." *Scientific Reports*, 6, (March 2016): 1–16. https://doi.org/10.1038/srep23580.

Rand, William Lee. *An Evidence-Based History of Reiki: A Selection of Articles from Reiki News Magazine.* Southfield, MI: International Center for Reiki Training, 2015.

———. "What Is the History of Reiki?" International Center for Reiki Training. Accessed March 1, 2018. www.reiki.org/faq/historyofreiki.html.

Streich, Marianne. "The Story of Dr. Chujiro Hayashi." *Reiki News Magazine*, September 2009. https://www.reikimembership.com/ArticlesForms/Hayashi.pdf.

Glossary

attunement: The process in which a Reiki master-teacher aligns a Reiki student with Reiki healing energy and symbols

aura: The energetic field surrounding living beings

chakra: An energy center that connects body to mind and spirit

Chiryo: Treatment, moving the hands to where the Reiki energy is needed; one of the three pillars of Reiki

Cho Ku Rei (CKR): The Reiki power symbol

Dai Ko Myo (DKM): The Reiki master symbol

first-degree Reiki: The first degree of Reiki healing a practitioner is attuned to for hands-on healing

Gassho: A Reiki meditation practice involving holding both hands in prayer position and focusing on where the fingertips of the middle fingers touch; one of the three pillars of Reiki

Hara: The energetic center of the being and the primary connection point between the physical and the etheric located behind the belly button

Hon Sha Ze Sho Nen (HSZN): The Reiki distance symbol

meridian: An energetic pathway in humans

prana: Life force energy (also called qi)

Reiji Ho: Using an intuitive process to determine where energetic imbalances exist in the client; one of the three pillars of Reiki

Reiki: Universal healing energy

second-degree Reiki: The second degree of Reiki healing a practitioner is attuned to, which includes the second-degree Reiki symbols for distance healing, emotional healing, and power

Sei He Ki (SHK): Mental/emotional Reiki symbol

third-degree Reiki: The highest degree of Reiki attunement; allows the Reiki practitioner to teach and attune others to Reiki energy (also called Reiki master-teacher)

Usui Ryoho Reiki: The form of Reiki healing brought to the West by Hawayo Takata, based on the teachings of Dr. Mikao Usui (also referred to as Usui Reiki)

Index

About the Author

KAREN FRAZIER is an intuitive energy healer, a metaphysical healer, an Usui Ryoho Reiki master-teacher, and a member of the International Association of Reiki Professionals. She is also an ordained metaphysical minister with the International Metaphysical Ministry; holds a bachelor's degree, a master's degree, and a PhD in metaphysics; and is currently working on earning her doctor of divinity (DD) in spiritual healing.

Karen is the health editor for the website LoveToKnow. She's the author of multiple books about energy healing, crystals, and dream interpretation, and she writes two columns about metaphysics and energy healing for *Paranormal Underground Magazine*. She teaches Reiki and energy healing classes in the Portland, Oregon, area and is the founder of the SHARe Reiki Community. Learn more on her website, www.authorkarenfrazier.com.

Printed in the USA
CPSIA information can be obtained
at www.ICGtesting.com
CBHW040447310524
9306CB00013B/209